T0383721

Ruth L. Hall, PhD
Carole A. Oglesby, PhD
Editors

Exercise and Sport in Feminist Therapy: Constructing Modalities and Assessing Outcomes

Exercise and Sport in Feminist Therapy: Constructing Modalities and Assessing Outcomes has been co-published simultaneously as *Women & Therapy*, Volume 25, Number 2 2002.

Pre-publication
REVIEWS,
COMMENTARIES,
EVALUATIONS . . .

"VERY READABLE AND INFORMATIVE . . . EDUCATIONAL AND USEFUL, with practical applications for clinical practice as well as teaching. This is one of the first books to address the importance and impact of exercise and sport from a feminist perspective. In addition, it is GROUNDBREAKING in its attention to cultural and gender differences in exercise and sport, and their roles in psychological well-being. RECOMMENDED for clinicians who want to expand their repertoire of interventions for women, for those who are interested in exercise and sport, and for those interested in the integration of feminist theory and sport psychology."

Connie S. Chan, PhD
Professor, College of Public and Community Service, University of Massachusetts–Boston

Exercise and Sport in Feminist Therapy: Constructing Modalities and Assessing Outcomes

Exercise and Sport in Feminist Therapy: Constructing Modalities and Assessing Outcomes has been co-published simultaneously as *Women & Therapy*, Volume 25, Number 2 2002.

The *Women & Therapy* Monographic "Separates"

Below is a list of "separates," which in serials librarianship means a special issue simultaneously published as a special journal issue or double-issue *and* as a "separate" hardbound monograph. (This is a format which we also call a "DocuSerial.")

"Separates" are published because specialized libraries or professionals may wish to purchase a specific thematic issue by itself in a format which can be separately cataloged and shelved, as opposed to purchasing the journal on an on-going basis. Faculty members may also more easily consider a "separate" for classroom adoption.

"Separates" are carefully classified separately with the major book jobbers so that the journal tie-in can be noted on new book order slips to avoid duplicate purchasing.

You may wish to visit Haworth's website at . . .

http://www.HaworthPress.com

. . . to search our online catalog for complete tables of contents of these separates and related publications.

You may also call 1-800-HAWORTH (outside US/Canada: 607-722-5857), or Fax 1-800-895-0582 (outside US/Canada: 607-771-0012), or e-mail at:

getinfo@haworthpressinc.com

Exercise and Sport in Feminist Therapy: Constructing Modalities and Assessing Outcomes, edited by Ruth L. Hall, PhD, and Carole A. Oglesby, PhD (Vol. 25, No. 2, 2002). *Explores the healing use of exercise and sport as a helpful adjunct to feminist therapy.*

The Invisible Alliance: Psyche and Spirits in Feminist Therapy, edited by Ellyn Kaschak, PhD (Vol. 24, No. 3/4, 2001). *The richness of this volume is reflected in the diversity of the collected viewpoints, perspectives, and practices.. Each chapter challenges us to move out of the confines of our traditional training and reflect on the importance of spirituality. This book also brings us back to the original meaning of psychology–the study and knowledge of the soul" (Stephanie S. Covington, PhD, LCSW, Co-Director, Institute for Relational Development, La Jolla, California; Author,* A Woman's Way Through the Twelve Steps)

A New View of Women's Sexual Problems, edited by Ellyn Kaschak, PhD, and Leonore Tiefer, PhD (Vol. 24, No. 1/2, 2001). *"This useful, complex, and valid critique of simplistic notions of women's sexuality will be especially valuable for women's studies and public health courses. An important compilation representing many diverse individuals and groups of women." (Judy Norsigian and Jane Pincus, Co-Founders, Boston Women's Health Collective; Co-Authors,* Our Bodies, Ourselves for the New Century)

Intimate Betrayal: Domestic Violence in Lesbian Relationships, edited by Ellyn Kaschak, PhD (Vol. 23, No. 3, 2001). *"A groundbreaking examination of a taboo and complex subject. Both scholarly and down to earth, this superbly edited volume is an indispensable resource for clinicians, researchers, and lesbians caught up in the cycle of domestic violence." (Dr. Marny Hall, Psychotherapist; Author of* The Lesbian Love Companion, *Co-Author of* Queer Blues)

The Next Generation: Third Wave Feminist Psychotherapy, edited by Ellyn Kaschak, PhD (Vol. 23, No. 2, 2001). *Discusses the issues young feminists face, focusing on the implications for psychotherapists of the false sense that feminism is no longer necessary.*

Minding the Body: Psychotherapy in Cases of Chronic and Life-Threatening Illness, edited by Ellyn Kaschak, PhD (Vol. 23, No. 1, 2001). *Being diagnosed with cancer, lupus, or fibromyalgia is a traumatic event. All too often, women are told their disease is 'all in their heads' and therefore both 'unreal and insignificant' by a medical profession that dismisses emotions and scorns mental illness. Combining personal narratives and theoretical views of illness,* Minding the Body *offers an alternative approach to the mind-body connection. This book shows the reader how to deal with the painful and difficult emotions that exacerbate illness, while learning the emotional and spiritual lessons illness can teach.*

For Love or Money: The Fee in Feminist Therapy, edited by Marcia Hill, EdD, and Ellyn Kaschak, PhD (Vol. 22, No. 3, 1999). *"Recommended reading for both new and seasoned professionals . . . . An exciting and timely book about 'the last taboo' . . . . " (Carolyn C. Larsen, PhD, Senior Counsellor Emeritus, University of Calgary; Partner, Alberta Psychological Resources Ltd., Calgary, and Co-editor,* Ethical Decision Making in Therapy: Feminist Perspectives)

Beyond the Rule Book: Moral Issues and Dilemmas in the Practice of Psychotherapy, edited by Ellyn Kaschak, PhD, and Marcia Hill, EdD (Vol. 22, No. 2, 1999). *"The authors in this important and timely book tackle the difficult task of working through . . . conflicts, sharing their moral struggles and real life solutions in working with diverse populations and in a variety of clinical settings. . . . Will provide psychotherapists with a thought-provoking source for the stimulating and essential discussion of our own and our profession's moral bases." (Carolyn C. Larsen, PhD, Senior Counsellor Emeritus, University of Calgary, Partner in private practice, Alberta Psychological Resources Ltd., Calgary, and Co-editor,* Ethical Decision Making in Therapy: Feminist Perspectives)

Assault on the Soul: Women in the Former Yugoslavia, edited by Sara Sharratt, PhD, and Ellyn Kaschak, PhD (Vol. 22, No. 1, 1999). *Explores the applications and intersections of feminist therapy, activism and jurisprudence with women and children in the former Yugoslavia.*

Learning from Our Mistakes: Difficulties and Failures in Feminist Therapy, edited by Marcia Hill, EdD, and Esther D. Rothblum, PhD (Vol. 21, No. 3, 1998). *"A courageous and fundamental step in evolving a well-grounded body of theory and of investigating the assumptions that unexamined, lead us to error." (Teresa Bernardez, MD, Training and Supervising Analyst, The Michigan Psychoanalytic Council)*

Feminist Therapy as a Political Act, edited by Marcia Hill, EdD (Vol. 21, No. 2, 1998). *"A real contribution to the field. . . . A valuable tool for feminist therapists and those who want to learn about feminist therapy." (Florence L. Denmark, PhD, Robert S. Pace Distinguished Professor of Psychology and Chair, Psychology Department, Pace University, New York, New York)*

Breaking the Rules: Women in Prison and Feminist Therapy, edited by Judy Harden, PhD, and Marcia Hill, EdD (Vol. 20, No. 4 & Vol. 21, No. 1, 1998). *"Fills a long-recognized gap in the psychology of women curricula, demonstrating that feminist theory can be made relevant to the practice of feminism, even in prison." (Suzanne J. Kessler, PhD, Professor of Psychology and Women's Studies, State University of New York at Purchase)*

Children's Rights, Therapists' Responsibilities: Feminist Commentaries, edited by Gail Anderson, MA, and Marcia Hill, EdD (Vol. 20, No. 2, 1997). *"Addresses specific practice dimensions that will help therapists organize and resolve conflicts about working with children, adolescents, and their families in therapy." (Feminist Bookstore News)*

More than a Mirror: How Clients Influence Therapists' Lives, edited by Marcia Hill, EdD (Vol. 20, No. 1, 1997). *"Courageous, insightful, and deeply moving. These pages reveal the scrupulous self-examination and self-reflection of conscientious therapists at their best. An important contribution to feminist therapy literature and a book worth reading by therapists and clients alike." (Rachel Josefowitz Siegal, MSW, retired feminist therapy practitioner; Co-Editor,* Women Changing Therapy; Jewish Women in Therapy; *and* Celebrating the Lives of Jewish Women: Patterns in a Feminist Sampler)

Sexualities, edited by Marny Hall, PhD, LCSW (Vol. 19, No. 4, 1997). *"Explores the diverse and multifaceted nature of female sexuality, covering topics including sadomasochism in the therapy room, sexual exploitation in cults, and genderbending in cyberspace." (Feminist Bookstore News)*

Couples Therapy: Feminist Perspectives, edited by Marcia Hill, EdD, and Esther D. Rothblum, PhD (Vol. 19, No. 3, 1996). *Addresses some of the inadequacies, omissions, and assumptions in traditional couples' therapy to help you face the issues of race, ethnicity, and sexual orientation in helping couples today.*

A Feminist Clinician's Guide to the Memory Debate, edited by Susan Contratto, PhD, and M. Janice Gutfreund, PhD (Vol. 19, No. 1, 1996). *"Unites diverse scholars, clinicians, and activists in an insightful and useful examination of the issues related to recovered memories." (Feminist Bookstore News)*

Classism and Feminist Therapy: Counting Costs, edited by Marcia Hill, EdD, and Esther D. Rothblum, PhD (Vol. 18, No. 3/4, 1996). *"Educates, challenges, and questions the influence of classism on the clinical practice of psychotherapy with women." (Kathleen P. Gates, MA, Certified Professional Counselor, Center for Psychological Health, Superior, Wisconsin)*

Lesbian Therapists and Their Therapy: From Both Sides of the Couch, edited by Nancy D. Davis, MD, Ellen Cole, PhD, and Esther D. Rothblum, PhD (Vol. 18, No. 2, 1996). *"Highlights the power and boundary issues of psychotherapy from perspectives that many readers may have neither considered nor experienced in their own professional lives." (Psychiatric Services)*

Feminist Foremothers in Women's Studies, Psychology, and Mental Health, edited by Phyllis Chesler, PhD, Esther D. Rothblum, PhD, and Ellen Cole, PhD (Vol. 17, No. 1/2/3/4, 1995). *"A must for feminist scholars and teachers . . . These women's personal experiences are poignant and powerful." (Women's Studies International Forum)*

Women's Spirituality, Women's Lives, edited by Judith Ochshorn, PhD, and Ellen Cole, PhD (Vol. 16, No. 2/3, 1995). *"A delightful and complex book on spirituality and sacredness in women's lives." (Joan Clingan, MA, Spiritual Psychology, Graduate Advisor, Prescott College Master of Arts Program)*

Psychopharmacology from a Feminist Perspective, edited by Jean A. Hamilton, MD, Margaret Jensvold, MD, Esther D. Rothblum, PhD, and Ellen Cole, PhD (Vol. 16, No. 1, 1995). *"Challenges readers to increase their sensitivity and awareness of the role of sex and gender in response to and acceptance of pharmacologic therapy." (American Journal of Pharmaceutical Education)*

Wilderness Therapy for Women: The Power of Adventure, edited by Ellen Cole, PhD, Esther D. Rothblum, PhD, and Eve Erdman, MEd, MLS (Vol. 15, No. 3/4, 1994). *"There's an undeniable excitement in these pages about the thrilling satisfaction of meeting challenges in the physical world, the world outside our cities that is unfamiliar, uneasy territory for many women. If you're interested at all in the subject, this book is well worth your time." (Psychology of Women Quarterly)*

Bringing Ethics Alive: Feminist Ethics in Psychotherapy Practice, edited by Nanette K. Gartrell, MD (Vol. 15, No. 1, 1994). *"Examines the theoretical and practical issues of ethics in feminist therapies. From the responsibilities of training programs to include social issues ranging from racism to sexism to practice ethics, this outlines real questions and concerns." (Midwest Book Review)*

Women with Disabilities: Found Voices, edited by Mary Willmuth, PhD, and Lillian Holcomb, PhD (Vol. 14, No. 3/4, 1994). *"These powerful chapters often jolt the anti-disability consciousness and force readers to contend with the ways in which disability has been constructed, disguised, and rendered disgusting by much of society." (Academic Library Book Review)*

Faces of Women and Aging, edited by Nancy D. Davis, MD, Ellen Cole, PhD, and Esther D. Rothblum, PhD (Vol. 14, No. 1/2, 1993). *"This uplifting, helpful book is of great value not only for aging women, but also for women of all ages who are interested in taking active control of their own lives." (New Mature Woman)*

Refugee Women and Their Mental Health: Shattered Societies, Shattered Lives, edited by Ellen Cole, PhD, Oliva M. Espin, PhD, and Esther D. Rothblum, PhD (Vol. 13, No. 1/2/3, 1992). *"The ideas presented are rich and the perspectives varied, and the book is an important contribution to understanding refugee women in a global context." (Contemporary Psychology)*

Women, Girls and Psychotherapy: Reframing Resistance, edited by Carol Gilligan, PhD, Annie Rogers, PhD, and Deborah Tolman, EdD (Vol. 11, No. 3/4, 1991). *"Of use to educators, psychotherapists, and parents–in short, to any person who is directly involved with girls at adolescence." (Harvard Educational Review)*

Professional Training for Feminist Therapists: Personal Memoirs, edited by Esther D. Rothblum, PhD, and Ellen Cole, PhD (Vol. 11, No. 1, 1991). *"Exciting, interesting, and filled with the angst and the energies that directed these women to develop an entirely different approach to counseling." (Science Books & Films)*

Monographs "Separates" list continued at the back

Exercise and Sport in Feminist Therapy: Constructing Modalities and Assessing Outcomes

Ruth L. Hall, PhD
Carole A. Oglesby, PhD
Editors

Exercise and Sport in Feminist Therapy: Constructing Modalities and Assessing Outcomes has been co-published simultaneously as *Women & Therapy*, Volume 25, Number 2 2002.

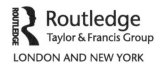

Routledge
Taylor & Francis Group

LONDON AND NEW YORK

Exercise and Sport in Feminist Therapy: Constructing Modalities and Assessing Outcomes has been co-published simultaneously as *Women & Therapy*™, Volume 25, Number 2 2002.

First published 2002 by The Haworth Press, Inc.

2 Park Square, Milton Park, Abingdon, Oxfordshire OX14 4RN
605 Third Avenue, New York, NY 10017

Routledge is an imprint of the Taylor & Francis Group, an informa business

First issued in hardback 2020

Cover design by Marylouise E. Doyle

Library of Congress Cataloging-in-Publication Data

Exercise and sport in feminist therapy : constructing modalities and assessing outcomes / Ruth L. Hall, Carole A. Oglesby, editors.
    p. cm.
"Co-published simultaneously as Women & Therapy, Volume 25, Number 2 2002."
    1. Feminist therapy. 2. Sports–Psychological aspects. 3. Exercise–Psychological aspects. 4. Sports for women. 5. Exercise for women. I. Hall, Ruth L. (Ruth Louise) II. Oglesby, Carole A. III. Women & therapy.
RC489.F45 E94 2002
615.8'2'082–dc21

                                                                      2002005920

ISBN 13: 978-0-7890-1912-7 (hbk)
ISBN 13: 978-0-7890-1913-4 (pbk)

Indexing, Abstracting & Website/Internet Coverage

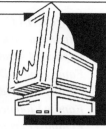

This section provides you with a list of major indexing & abstracting services. That is to say, each service began covering this periodical during the year noted in the right column. Most Websites which are listed below have indicated that they will either post, disseminate, compile, archive, cite or alert their own Website users with research-based content from this work. (This list is as current as the copyright date of this publication.)

(continued)

(continued)

Special Bibliographic Notes related to special journal issues (separates) and indexing/abstracting:

- indexing/abstracting services in this list will also cover material in any "separate" that is co-published simultaneously with Haworth's special thematic journal issue or DocuSerial. Indexing/abstracting usually covers material at the article/chapter level.
- monographic co-editions are intended for either non-subscribers or libraries which intend to purchase a second copy for their circulating collections.
- monographic co-editions are reported to all jobbers/wholesalers/approval plans. The source journal is listed as the "series" to assist the prevention of duplicate purchasing in the same manner utilized for books-in-series.
- to facilitate user/access services all indexing/abstracting services are encouraged to utilize the co-indexing entry note indicated at the bottom of the first page of each article/chapter/contribution.
- this is intended to assist a library user of any reference tool (whether print, electronic, online, or CD-ROM) to locate the monographic version if the library has purchased this version but not a subscription to the source journal.
- individual articles/chapters in any Haworth publication are also available through the Haworth Document Delivery Service (HDDS).

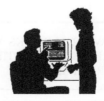

Exercise and Sport in Feminist Therapy: Constructing Modalities and Assessing Outcomes

CONTENTS

ABOUT THE EDITORS

Ruth L. Hall, PhD, is a licensed psychologist and Associate Professor in the Department of Psychology at The College of New Jersey. She also maintains a private practice and consults to various agencies and organizations. She received her PhD in clinical/community psychology from Boston University and her MEd in sport psychology from Temple University. Dr. Hall is a member of the Women's Sports Foundation Advisory Board. Her publications and presentations primarily address people of color, women, and athletes. A recent publication, *Mind and Body: Toward the Holistic Treatment of African-American Women*, received the Association for Women in Psychology's (AWP) Women of Color Psychologies Award. She is also an associate editor of *The Encyclopedia of Women and Sport in America*. In 1995, Dr. Hall received the AWP's Christine Ladd-Franklin Award for outstanding service to the AWP and to feminist psychology. She is a Fellow of the American Psychological Association and former president of Section One (Black Women) of APA's Division 35. Dr. Hall is a certified sport psychologist.

Carole A. Oglesby, PhD, has been Professor of Kinesiology at Temple University since 1975. She has published extensively and is the senior editor of *The Encyclopedia of Women and Sport in America*. She was Health and Exercise Psychology Chairperson for the Association for the Advancement of Applied Sport Psychology (AAASP) and AAASP's first liaison to Division 38 (Health Psychology) of the American Psychological Association. Dr. Oglesby is also certified as a sport psychology consultant by AAASP. She is on the registry of sport-psychology consultants maintained by the United States Olympic Committee and is President of WomenSport International.

INTRODUCTION

Ruth L. Hall
Carole A. Oglesby

In the arena of psychological health, there continues to be a critical need for overall mental health planning for women and the implementation of women-centered services. Halbreich (1998) stated that gender and gender bias still influence women's socioeconomic interactions, mental, physical and economic health and that environmental stressors are fundamental influences in women's mental health challenges. As a result of these and other factors, data reveal that the psychological health of women is often compromised. The magnitude of mental and physical illness in women, both personally and on a societal basis, is immense. Murray and Lopez (1996) report that mental disorders are the second leading cause of disability among the world's women and predict that by 2020, they will be the leading cause. Further, women experience more depression, anxiety and panic disorders, rapid cycling bipolar disorders and eating disorders than men. Yonkers (1998) stated that the predominance of unipolar mood disorders in women is one of the most stable and widely replicated findings in psychiatry. A recent survey of over 8,000 individuals in the United States, from a wide variety of socioeconomic levels, revealed a lifetime prevalence of major depressive disorders in 21% of women and 13% of men. These data parallel an international survey conducted in Germany, Canada

[Haworth co-indexing entry note]: "Introduction." Hall, Ruth L., and Carole A. Oglesby. Co-published simultaneously in *Women & Therapy* (The Haworth Press, Inc.) Vol. 25, No. 2, 2002, pp. 1-7; and: *Exercise and Sport in Feminist Therapy: Constructing Modalities and Assessing Outcomes* (ed: Ruth L. Hall, and Carole A. Oglesby) The Haworth Press, Inc., 2002, pp. 1-7. Single or multiple copies of this article are available for a fee from The Haworth Document Delivery Service [1-800-HAWORTH, 9:00 a.m. - 5:00 p.m. (EST). E-mail address: getinfo@haworthpressinc.com].

1

and New Zealand revealing a 2:1 ratio in mood disorders when comparing women to men (Yonkers, 1998).

In general, cultural differences are frequently ignored in diagnosis, and instruments that assess psychopathology are not normed on culturally diverse populations. This pattern leads to misdiagnosis, particularly among women (Matsumoto, 2000; Messich, Kleinman, Fabrega, & Parton, 1996).

Quietly co-existing with the body of evidence of women's vulnerabilities in the areas of mental health, has been accumulating evidence, in sport and exercise science and in medical epidemiology, concerning the health benefits of active lifestyle (Berger, 1996). In the general population, planned/structured physical activity has been associated with benefits in four broad areas: enhanced mood (Steptoe & Cox, 1988; Berger, 1996; Berger & Motl, 2000), stress reduction, positive self concept (Soenstroem,1998), and higher quality of life (Donahue, 1994; Berger, 1996). The psychological benefits appear to be even more pronounced among special populations such as clinically depressed and anxious clients, cardiac patients, the elderly and others with specific diseases (Berger, 1996). Although the research is not extensive among clinical populations, the improvement in mood following exercise has been demonstrated in acute (Nelson & Morgan, 1994; Feldman, 1995) and chronic clinical populations (Martinson, 1993; Martinson & Morgan, 1997).

Physical activity participation has demonstrated potential in mediating the impact of child sexual abuse on the resilience of adult women. Researchers identified three contexts of achievement which gave girls opportunities to experience success and healing; academics, social activities and sport (Romans, Martins, Anderson, O'Shea, & Mullen, 1995). Stuhlmiller (1994) has also described the helpful role of so-called "action therapies" in work with female clients suffering from post traumatic stress disorder.

Moreover, exercise programs have demonstrated the capacity to reduce falls, improve muscle strength, size and flexibility, and reduce depression in the elderly (Halfant, 1998). These results, from a 1993 National Institute of Aging multi-site study, held true for samples ranging from community centers to retirement and nursing homes, with age ranges of participants from 60-90. Halfant also suggests that exercise is as effective in maintaining a healthy lifestyle for elders as for any other age cohort.

Halbreich (1998) affirms a recognized truism that women's mental health is an inter-disciplinary field and involves a variety of experts from disciplines including mental health specialists, researchers from the social and natural sciences, medical specialists including gynecologists, endocrinologists, neuroscientists, and advocacy organizations. Conspicuously absent in this recitation is any explicit recognition of sport and exercise science and its contribution to women's health. The integration of sport/exercise regimens as adjuncts to treatment in psychology training programs is rare, especially for female clients. The failure to embrace sport/exercise habits as "natural" concomitants of healthy functioning is, undoubtedly, rooted in the same soil that creates other unhealthy conditions of women's lives.

It is beyond the scope of this volume to address the matter of the relation of women to sport and physicality. There is an extensive treatment of this phenomenon in several sport sociology and psychology texts (Oglesby, 1978; Birrell & Coles, 1994; Cohen, 2001). One of the core issues of the limitation of women is expressed in Spears' (1978) delineation of the "cult of true womanhood" which dominated discussions of white women in the 19th and early 20th centuries.

> Their homes demonstrated their inability to perform useful tasks or engage in physical activity beyond the occasional game of croquet. The fragile female remained the epitome of womanhood . . . delicacy was desired and ill-health their fate. (p. 8)

Scientific, educational and advocacy efforts of the past 30 years have been particularly focused on overturning this legacy but the battle cannot be claimed as won. For example, the World Health Organization (Mental Health Departments and Populations, 2000) suggests that poor women, in particular, may find it difficult to cope effectively. Due to environmental and educational barriers, illness and stress prevention strategies such as proper exercise and nutrition, accessing mental health services, moving to safer areas, saving money and effective use of discretionary time are difficult to enact. Clearly, the poor, and by implication, a disproportionate number of women of color are not "protected" but are still deprived of the benefits of exercise. Poor and/or rural women and women of color have had little if any opportunity to live a leisure-based lifestyle and physical labor, racism, classism and cultural and religious considerations drain away the possibility of a self-chosen active lifestyle (Hall, 1998; Corbett, 2000; Green, 2000; Pittman, 1999).

Yet another barrier to the full integration of sport/exercise as a recognized adjunct to therapy is the tradition of dualism, the mind-body split so pervasive in Western thought. This separation has a long and distinguished history in mental health where the focus has been on cognitive/emotional processes as the sole venue of change. Feminists and feminist therapists have confronted the flawed thinking of asking women to fit into stifling social roles in order to be "mentally healthy." Instead, we have strongly urged women to empower (and embody) themselves and to challenge the system invested in maintaining the status quo. This volume pushes the envelope further by asking women to challenge limiting cognitive assumptions about being women AND to reclaim their bodies in a healthful manner.

We maintain that holistic psychotherapeutic process, as described here, will proceed best if the theory and practice of psychology is integrated with the knowledge and approaches toward sport and exercise explicated in Kinesiology and Physical Education. The sub-disciplines of this domain (sport psychology, athletic training, motor control) have long focused on the challenge of maintaining active lifestyle for everyone, especially women. A phenomenon has been recognized and identified as "the exercise dilemma" whereby so many are benefited but so few participate (Berger, 1996). It is estimated that 9% of Americans exercise appropriately and more than 30% are completely sedentary (Berger, 1996).

It is not sufficient to give information on health risks and benefits of exercise nor to simply encourage and exhort exercise as a critical component of holistic/mental health. This approach has been attempted for generations by devotees among physical educators, therapists and physicians. Berger and Motl's (2000) extensive research suggests some of the deeper considerations embedded in behavior changes underlying active lifestyle:

1. The importance of discovery and delineation of one's personal meaning for sport/exercise. Meanings are unique to the individual and may range across intentions such as pursuit of flow or Zen state, burning calories, looking/feeling good, body-building, increasing self-esteem and being with friends and loved ones.

2. Finding a physical activity that is enjoyable. No pain-no gain probably holds "no truth" for most of us. Participation tends to be maintained in situations in which the experience is pleasant to one's sensibilities. The variety of physical activities is virtually infinite and new movement/sport forms are being created all the time (e.g., water aerobics). One must take the time and have the " know how" to experiment with the perspective of identifying an optimal match between client and movement activity of choice.

3. Recognize that all sport/exercise forms are not alike in modal requirements and only some modes seem consistently to aid in meeting goals like the alleviation of depression and anxiety. For example, activity that provides rhythmic breathing (walking/jogging, swimming), the relative absence of interpersonal competition, and is "closed" or repetitive motion (walking, swimming,

hatha yoga, or bowling in a recreation-oriented setting) is best suited for mood disorders.

4. Establish patterns of optimal frequency/intensity. With mood enhancement goals, research supports the practice of regular (3-5 times/week) and/or scheduled bouts of exercise, at a moderate intensity for 20-30 minutes minimum.

The authors in this volume display a diversity of theory and research approaches, including the integration of the exercise/sport sciences and exercise physiology. These contributors speak from a special appreciation of the concrete, physiological realities of the body. Sport/exercise habits, for them, are impacted by parameters of cardio-vascular endurance levels and degrees of flexibility along with phenomena such as subjectively held perceptions of capability. The inter-disciplinary teams, envisioned in our "new day" of holistic health professionals, can be enriched by inclusion of these vantage points. As clinicians and sport/exercise psychologists and consultants, we have sought to create a volume illustrating the interface of traditional mental and physical components of health. This volume is unique in that there is comparatively little written about the use of exercise in therapy even though, as these authors attest, exercise is a wonderful/useful intervention tool with depression, stress management, anxiety disorders and chronic pain management. They illustrate how exercise can be applied to inpatient and outpatient populations, to the neurotic and the chronically mentally ill. Exercise can reduce the incidence of chronic diseases, including diabetes and hypertension, as well as address physical problems such as obesity. Exercise can give one a sense of mastery and self-confidence. Since exercise is so effective with such a broad range of clients with a wide range of symptoms and diagnoses, it is surprising that it is not used more consistently with clients. As our authors suggest, exercise must be tailored to specific issues and client populations and diagnosis, level of functioning, age, overall health and a cultural context must be taken into account.

One of the challenges reflected in all the writings is that of instituting an exercise regimen and the need for a support structure available to the client. Clearly, more research needs to be done and more needs to be written about exercise and therapy. This is a beginning, and we hope that this volume will not only encourage other therapists to write about using exercise in therapy but will encourage more therapists and clients to appreciate exercise and integrate exercise into their lifestyle.

REFERENCES

Berger, B. (1996). Psychological benefits of an active lifestyle: What we know and what we need to know. *Quest, 48*, 330-353.

Berger, B., & Motl, R. (2000). Exercise and mood: A selective review and synthesis of research employing the profile of mood states. *Journal of Athletics and Sport Psychology, 12*, 69-92.

Birrell, S. & Coles, C. (1994). Women, sport and culture. Champaign, IL: Human Kinetics.

Cohen, G. (2001). *Women and sport: Issues and controversies*. Oxen Hill, MD: AAHPERD Publications.

Corbett, D. (2000). The African American female in collegiate sport: Racism and sexism. In D. Brooks, & R. Althouse (Eds.), *Racism in collegiate athletics*, pp. 196-226. Morgantown, WV: Fitness Information Technology.

Donahue, B. (1994). The way of the warrior: One metaphor for individuation. In M. Stein & J. Hollwitz (Eds.), *Psyche and sports* (pp. 89-109). Wilmette, IL: Chiron.

Feldman, L. (1995). Variations in circumplex structure of mood. *Personality and Social Psychology Bulletin, 21*, 806-817.

Green, T. (2000). The future of the African American female athlete. In D. Brooks & R. Althouse (Eds.), *Racism in collegiate sports* (pp. 227-244) Morgantown, WV: Fitness Information Technology.

Halbreich, U. (1998). Evaluation of women's mental health: Delineation of the field, and needs and steps toward a consensus. *Psychopharmacology Bulletin, 34*(3), 247-249.

Halfant, M. (1998). Exercise and elderly women. In C. Oglesby (Ed.), *Encyclopedia of women and sport in America* (pp. 85-86) Phoenix, AZ: Oryx.

Hall, R. L. (1998). Mind and body: Toward the holistic treatment of African American women. *The Psychotherapy Patient, 10* (3/4), 81-100.

Martinson, E. (1993). Therapeutic implications of exercise for clinically anxious and depressed patients. *International Journal of Sport Psychology, 24*, 185-199.

Martinson, E., & Morgan, W. (1997). Antidepressant effects of physical activity. In W. P. Morgan (Ed.), *Physical activity and mental health* (pp. 93-106). Washington, DC: Taylor and Francis.

Matsumoto, D. (2000). *Culture and psychology: People around the world* (2nd ed.). Belmont, CA: Wadsworth.

Mental Health Determinants and Populations, Department of Mental Health and Substance Dependence. (2000). *Women's mental health: An evidence based review*. World Health Organization: Geneva, Switzerland.

Messich, J. E., Kleinman, A., Fabrega, H. & Parton, F. (1996). *Culture and psychiatric diagnosis: A DSM-IV perspective*. Washington, DC: American Psychiatric Press, Inc.

Murray, C., & Lopez, A. (1996). *The global burden of disease*. Cambridge, MA: Harvard University Press.

Nelson, T., & Morgan, W. (1994). Acute effects of exercise on mood in depressed female students. *Medicine and Science in Sport and Exercise, 26*, S156.

Oglesby, C. (1978). *Women and sport: From myth to reality*. Philadelphia, PA: Lea & Febiger.

Pittman, B. (1999). *A qualitative study of beauty standards in the African American community*. Unpublished research study, Department of Kinesiology, Temple University, Philadelphia, PA.

Romans, S., Martins, J., Anderson, J., O'Shea, M., & Mullen, P. (1995). Factors that mediate between child sexual abuse and adult psychological outcome. *Psychological Medicine, 25*, 127-145.

Sonstroem, R. (1981). Exercise and self-esteem: Recommendations for expository research. *Quest, 33*, 124-139.

Spears, B. (1978). The myth. In C. Oglesby (Ed.), *Women and sport: From myth to reality*. (pp. 2-12) Philadelphia, PA: Lea & Febiger.

Steptoe, A., & Cox, S. (1988). Acute effects of exercise on mood. *Health Psychology, 7*, 329-340.

Stuhlmiller, C. (1994). Action-based therapy for post-traumatic stress disorder. In M. B. Williams & J. F. Sommer, Jr. (Eds.), *Handbook of post traumatic therapy* (pp. 386-400) Westport, CT: Greenwood.

Yonkers, K. (1998). Assessing unipolar mood disorders in women. *Psychopharmacology Bulletin*, 34(3), 261-266.

THEORY APPROACHES
FROM PSYCHOLOGY

Can Exercise Contribute to the Goals
of Feminist Therapy?

Joan C. Chrisler
Jean M. Lamont

SUMMARY. Exercise can contribute to the feminist therapy goals of empowerment and consciousness raising, and it can help to alleviate depression, manage stress, reduce anxiety, improve body image, raise self-esteem and self-efficacy, and aid recovery from physical or sexual abuse. The purposes of this article are to review the potential contributions of exercise to feminist therapy and to encourage therapists to consider how their clients could benefit from engagement in regular physical exercise. *[Article copies available for a fee from The Haworth Document Delivery Service: 1-800-HAWORTH. E-mail address: <getinfo@ haworthpressinc.com> Website: <http://www.HaworthPress.com> © 2002 by The Haworth Press, Inc. All rights reserved.]*

Joan C. Chrisler and Jean M. Lamont are affiliated with Connecticut College.
Address correspondence to: Joan C. Chrisler, PhD, Department of Psychology, Connecticut College, New London, CT 06320 (E-mail: jcchr@conncoll.edu).

[Haworth co-indexing entry note]: "Can Exercise Contribute to the Goals of Feminist Therapy?" Chrisler, Joan C., and Jean M. Lamont. Co-published simultaneously in *Women & Therapy* (The Haworth Press, Inc.) Vol. 25, No. 2, 2002, pp. 9-22; and: *Exercise and Sport in Feminist Therapy: Constructing Modalities and Assessing Outcomes* (ed: Ruth L. Hall, and Carole A. Oglesby) The Haworth Press, Inc., 2002, pp. 9-22. Single or multiple copies of this article are available for a fee from The Haworth Document Delivery Service [1-800-HAWORTH, 9:00 a.m. - 5:00 p.m. (EST). E-mail address: getinfo@haworthpressinc.com].

KEYWORDS. Feminist therapy, exercise, women

"In the battle for equality, women need strong bodies as well as quick minds."

–Susan B. Anthony, c. 1880

Susan B. Anthony (known as "Aunt Susan" to her colleagues in the movement for women's suffrage) often included in her speeches and writings an admonition to women to develop their strength, which she knew would be needed in what she believed (correctly) would be a long struggle for equal rights. It is clear that she meant for us to develop both physical and psychological strength. Physical strength gives us the stamina we need to persist toward our goals; psychological strength gives us the resilience we need to recover from the inevitable setbacks along the way. We think her advice is as relevant in the 21st century as it was in the 19th.

Feminist therapists have written a great deal about women's psychological strength and techniques for enhancing it. However, relatively little attention has been paid to the importance of women's physical fitness. Perhaps this is a generational issue; as more post-Title IX women begin writing about psychotherapy, exercise may assume more importance. Or perhaps physical exercise and feminist therapy just don't seem to have much in common. Our academic and clinical work in health psychology lead us to believe that regular physical exercise can contribute to the goals of feminist therapy. We hope to convince you to agree.

WHAT IS FEMINIST THERAPY?

Feminist therapy is difficult to define because it does not endorse a specific set of therapeutic techniques, as do other forms of therapy (e.g., psychoanalysis, behavior therapy, cognitive therapy). It can be thought of as psychotherapy illuminated by feminist political theory. What makes therapy feminist is how therapists think about what they do, what types of problems they address, and the underlying feminist theoretical models that inform the practice (Brown, 1994). These philosophical matters are much more important than how the therapists work and which techniques they use.

Most feminist therapists agree on several defining principles: (a) the personal is political; (b) the importance of analyzing the contributions of power and gender to any social situation; (c) the need to bring women's own experiences from the margins to the center (Ballou & West, 2000; Brown, 1994; Worrel & Remer, 1992). It is also agreed that consciousness raising (CR) and empowerment are important goals of feminist therapy. Consciousness raising originated around 1970 as a political, educational, and organizing strategy, and one can think of CR groups as the precursors of feminist therapy. The purpose of CR is to learn about the connections between gender and power and then to become aware of how gender role expectations and political oppression have limited our behavior and personality, our goals and opportunities, indeed, most aspects of our lives and our selves. Unlike other therapies, feminist therapy will not help troubled or angry women to "fit in" to their roles more comfortably and quietly (Ballou & West, 2000). In fact, feminist therapy is considered most successful when it empowers women to "stand out" boldly and confidently in order to meet their own needs and to demand social and political changes that would make it easier for all women to define themselves.

Feminist therapy emphasizes both the similarity and the diversity among women, and it recognizes that gender is not the only dimension that requires a power analysis. There is a growing literature on feminist perspectives on power and class, race, sexual orientation, disability, illness, age, ethnicity, religion, body size, and other political categories. The post-modern notion of positionality is useful in feminist therapy; one must consider the location of each individual in the larger society and learn from them how the world looks from their life experiences.

Feminist therapists specialize in working on concerns and disorders that are common in women, both because of the belief that women's experiences should take priority and because of the more practical matter that most of their clients are women. Among the frequent foci of feminist therapy are depression, anxiety disorders, eating disorders, body image issues, relationship concerns, role conflicts, and sequelae of physical or sexual assault or abuse. Exercise can be a useful adjunct in therapy for any of these concerns.

WOMEN AND EXERCISE

It has been estimated that fewer than 10% of the adult American population meets the exercise guidelines recommended by the U.S. Surgeon General (King & Kiernan, 1997). Men's levels of physical activity are greater than women's at any age, but the gap widens as people grow older (Bassey, 2000), and ethnic minority women in the U.S. are even less physically active than European American women (King, Blair, Bild, Dishman, Duppert, Marcus, Oldridge, Paffenbarger, Powell, & Yeager,1992; Pate, Pratt, Blair, Haskell, Macera, Bouchard, Buchner, Caspersen, Ettinger, Heath, King, Kriska, Leon, Marcus, Morris, Paffenbarger, Patrick, Pollock, Rippe, Sallis, & Whitmore, 1995). Approximately 59% of all women in the U.S. are reported to be primarily sedentary; 65% of ethnic minority women are primarily sedentary (Pate et al.,1995). These statistics are troubling given the importance of exercise for physical and mental health. The risk of developing a number of chronic illnesses (e.g., hypertension, heart disease, diabetes, osteoporosis) can be lowered by engaging in regular physical activity (King & Kiernan, 1997; Light & Girdler, 1993). The statistics are also puzzling in light of the cultural messages we receive about the "health and fitness boom" that began in the 1970s. However, the group of women who have been most involved in fitness activities are circumscribed by class, culture, and generational cohort. Demographic predictors of a sedentary lifestyle include being older, female, and African American, and having less education, more body weight, and a history of being relatively physically inactive (Blair, Powell, Bazzarre, Early, Epstein, Green, Harris, Haskell, Ling, Koplan, Marcus, Paffenbarger, & Yeager, 1993).

A feminist analysis of women's negative or ambivalent attitudes toward exercise is instructive. Obviously, it is easier to control women and keep them in their proper sphere if they are physically weak and well aware of their lesser strength and undeveloped physical abilities. Many older women were brought up to believe that sports and exercise are fine for children but inappropriate for adult women. "Old-fashioned" beliefs that developing one's muscles or working up a sweat are unfeminine persist today not only in older women but in young women in some class and cultural groups (Hays, 1999; Nelson, 1998). Many girls have been actively discouraged from participating in team sports, and told that individual sports, especially those that emphasize gracefulness (e.g., gymnastics and figure skating) or involve the use of "light" objects (e.g., racquets), are more feminine than those that require physical force or the use of heavy objects (e.g., boats) (Mathes, 1978; Sage & Loudermilk, 1979; Snyder & Spreitzer, 1973). Prior to the enactment of Title IX, it was difficult for girls to find opportunities to participate in team sports even when they were motivated to do so. It's worth recalling that although Title IX went into effect in 1979, it suffered a serious setback after the 1984 Grove City v. Bell Supreme

Court decision, and was not fully reinstated until 1988 (Hall, 2000). The scarcity of role models, the dearth of facilities, the lack of attention to women's sports by the media, and insinuations that most female athletes and coaches are lesbians have also turned some girls away from sports and exercise (Nelson, 1998).

Many adult women who did not have much experience with sports and exercise in their youth have difficulty imagining that exercise can be fun. Instead they see it as work, as just another "should" in their busy lives (Hays, 1999). Research on psychosocial barriers to exercise most often identifies lack of interest and perceived (or expected) lack of enjoyment as the main barriers for women (Marcus, Dubbert, King, & Pinto, 1995). Social anxiety keeps some women away from exercise, especially those who are inexperienced, who cannot afford trendy exercise clothes and shoes, and who are obviously not physically fit or significantly exceed weight "standards" (O'Leary, 1992). Lack of free time due to heavy work and/or family role demands also keep women from exercising. Researchers have found that the presence of children in the home is the best predictor of women's inability to initiate or sustain an exercise program (Marcus, Pinto, Simkin, Audrain, & Taylor, 1994; Verhoef, Love, & Rose, 1992). Public spaces (e.g., parks, bicycle or jogging paths, playgrounds, streets) are not necessarily safe for women to use as exercise venues, and many women cannot afford to join exercise clubs, spas, or YWCAs, or pay for aerobics classes or swimming lessons at schools or community centers. The excessive concern about physical appearance that motivates some women to exercise compulsively keeps other women from exercising at all. Shame about body size and shape or embarrassment about clumsiness or lack of experience with athletic activities make some women reluctant to exercise in public spaces (Vertinsky, 1998). One cannot even walk briskly in fashionable clothes such as high heels and tight skirts, and women may be reluctant to work up a sweat that could interfere with expensive coiffures or cosmetics (Marcus et al., 1995). Finally, women may be anxious about breaking gender role constraints by dedicating themselves to a regular exercise routine because they are concerned that others will label them as selfish, competitive, ambitious, or masculine (Nelson, 1998).

RELEVANCE OF EXERCISE TO FEMINIST THERAPY

Exercise is relevant to many of the goals of feminist therapy. In addition to improving women's physical and mental health, exercise builds self-confidence and self-esteem, enhances self-efficacy, aids in stress management, serves as an object lesson in gender politics, and develops in women the stamina they need to work for social justice.

The Personal Is Political

The first lesson of consciousness raising is that what affects one woman always affects others, often many others. Rarely are our problems purely personal; depression, anxiety, stress, inequitable relationships, body dissatisfaction, and post-abuse or assault trauma are all examples of distress that is fundamentally political. All result from oppression due to sociocultural constraints that are designed to limit women's goals and opportunities and keep women in "their place." Women's ambivalence about exercise can be an object lesson to illustrate this concept. Individual women may say, "I just don't like exercise; I'm just not interested in sports." But how could they develop the interest when they grew up being told that sports were for men and that exercise is unfeminine, when there were few girls' teams available for them to join? Why should women be denied the fun and sense of freedom of movement that sports and exercise provide? Why shouldn't women gain strength and challenge their bodies? Why shouldn't we break gender role constraints? Redefine what it means to be a woman in a way that suits us? Own our bodies in positive ways?

Empowerment

Exercise is an obvious route to physical empowerment. Building cardiovascular fitness and developing muscles results in physical strength, stamina, and increased energy. Enhanced fitness and strength contribute to independence and well being as women find that they can do more things for themselves (e.g., carrying heavier loads, opening tight jars, walking farther). Self-strengthening also reinforces self-efficacy, the belief that one is able to do what one wants to do. Establishing an exercise routine is an accomplishment, especially for women who never thought they could do it. Clients can be helped to see that if they can make this lifestyle change, they can make as yet unimagined changes in their lives; if athletic skills can be acquired and developed, so can any others that they need for a better future.

Applications of Exercise to Mental Health

In addition to its relevance to overarching goals, exercise can be used as a specific therapy technique. It can be applied along with other therapeutic techniques to facilitate improvements in affect, reduction of body dissatisfaction, and recovery from trauma caused by physical or sexual assault or abuse.

Depression. There is an extensive empirical literature on the benefits of exercise. Among the best established benefits is the positive effect of exercise on mood. Many researchers (e.g., Berger & Owen, 1983, 1992; Doyne, Chambless, & Beutler, 1983; Hartz, Wallace, & Clayton, 1982; Joiner & Tickle, 1998; Nagy & Frazier, 1988) have found significant changes in scores on such measures as the Beck Depression Inventory and the Profile of Mood States in women who have engaged in regular (especially aerobic) exercise. Data from these studies also indicate decreases in fatigue, anger, tension, and confusion and increases in vigor, morale, self-esteem, internal locus of control, and global mood, all of which are related to depression. Among the types of exercise studied are aerobic routines, walking, line dancing, swimming, yoga, weight-lifting, racquetball, and running; all produced mood improvements. This list includes a variety of activities, some of which are suitable for women of all socioeconomic and ability levels. Aerobic "dance" routines can be done in one's living room and walking in one's neighborhood; they do not require expensive equipment. Weight-bearing exercises for the arms can be added gradually, beginning with the use of bags of beans or cans of soup. Non-impact exercise routines such as yoga and swimming are easier for elders who may have arthritic joints and low fitness levels. Therapists may want to recommend that clients find a friend to join them in their exercise plans. Social support increases the likelihood that lifestyle changes will be implemented and maintained, and the fun of being with a friend can also improve mood and serve as the main reinforcement until the exercise itself becomes fun (Hays, 1999; Minor & Brown, 1993). Furthermore, friends who exercise together are engaging in peer support and mutuality. They are taking care of themselves and each other in a way that self-in-relation theory predicts is comfortable for and valued by women (Gilligan, 1982; Jordan, Kaplan, Miller, Stiver, & Surrey, 1991; Miller, 1976).

Anxiety and Stress Reduction. Exercise is routinely recommended as a stress management technique because it provides an outlet for the energy that builds up as a result of the experience of stressors (racquetball and jogging may actually simulate "fight or flight responses"). Exercise also provides an opportunity to distract ourselves from the day's hassles and remove ourselves from the stressful environment. Runners' brains produce endorphins and other neurochemicals that have a calming and pain-reducing effect (Thoren, Floras, Hoffman, & Seals, 1990). Researchers have found that women who exercise regularly are less anxious and tense than those who do not (Joiner & Tickle, 1998; Nagy & Frazier, 1988; Norvell, Martin, & Salamon, 1991), that even one bout of exercise can reduce tension and improve mood (Pierce & Pate, 1994), and that people feel better and rate themselves more positively on days they exercise than on days they do not (Steptoe, Kimbell, & Basford, 1998). Exercise may improve sleep quality (Bazargan, 1996), which aids in reducing anxiety, and there is evidence that it reduces premenstrual tension and menstrual cramps (Choi, 1992; Steege & Blumenthal, 1993). Thus, exercise can be helpful in the treatment of anxiety disorders and in managing the stress caused by relationship conflicts or work and family role demands. Most life changes are stressful and may be accompanied by anxiety; exercise can help in coping with the affect that accompanies the experience of change.

Body Dissatisfaction. Body dissatisfaction is so common among women in the U.S. that it constitutes the norm (Rodin, Silberstein, & Striegel-Moore, 1985). Women are encouraged by advertisers of beauty products and by the popular press to believe that although they can never look good enough, the surest route to improving one's life is to change one's appearance (Malkin, Wornian, & Chrisler, 1999). Body image concerns can arise at any age (Chrisler & Ghiz, 1993; Flannery-Schroeder & Chrisler, 1996), and are not limited to body size and shape. Feminist therapists often use CR to show women that we have all been taught to see women's bodies as ornamental rather than instrumental (Saltzberg & Chrisler, 1995). Exercise can be useful in changing the focus from how one's body looks to how it works and what it can do. As they gain in fitness and stamina, women start to value their bodies' endurance, strength, and capabilities. Exercise also leads to heightened awareness of bodily sensations (Hays, 1994, 1999; Winborn, Myers, & Mulling, 1998), which may lead to a healthier type of body consciousness, including a greater ease with oneself, and has positive implications for general health and early disease detection. Obviously, exercise may result in changes in body weight and shape that make clients feel better about their bodies, but feminist therapists should place their emphasis on non-appearance-related benefits (e.g., prevention, energy) in order to avoid sanctioning the cultural messages that caused the body dissatisfaction to occur.

Eating Disorders. Body dissatisfaction, low self-esteem, and depression are predictors of eating disorders (Gardner, Stark, Friedman, & Jackson, 2000; Pettus, 2001). All can be improved by exercise; therefore, it is reasonable to assume that exercise is an important element of eating disorder prevention and can be helpful in the treatment of eating disorders. Regular exercise within reasonable limits is probably most beneficial in the treatment of compulsive eating and binge eating disorder. Therapists should take care to ascertain how much exercise clients with anorexia and bulimia are already doing. If exercise is an established purging technique, the plan should be to moderate existing routines to a healthy level rather than to encourage additional exercise. As we stated above, the focus should be changed from body weight and shape to physical health and strength. We know several former anorexics who have turned their obsession with weight into an obsession with nutrition (one is now a vegetarian) and turned from their compulsive calorie counting to daily exercise routines. Although their exercise is more rigid and purposeful than fun, they are now physically fit, healthy, and in the "standard" weight range (albeit at the low end) for their heights. One of the women is convinced that exercise has saved her life.

Sequelae of Physical and Sexual Assault and Abuse. Violence against women has psychological, sexual, and physical consequences. Depression, anxiety, and posttraumatic stress disorder are common in women who have experienced domestic violence, rape, and incest (Roades, 2000). We have already seen that exercise can ameliorate depression and anxiety. It can also help with PTSD signs and symptoms such as fear for safety, helplessness, sleep difficulties, and emotional numbing (Stuhlmiller, 1994). Martial arts training, which has frequently been encouraged as a step toward the prevention of assault (e.g., Bart & O'Brien, 1985; Rozee, 2000), may also be helpful in recovery from PTSD. In surveys (e.g., Eby, Campbell, Sullivan, & Davidson, 1995) of women who have experienced physical or sexual abuse as many as 50% report somatic complaints six months or more after the incidents. Among the common physical problems that exercise might help alleviate are: low energy, sleep problems, headaches, muscle tension or soreness, fatigue, weight change, back pain, poor appetite, and weakness. The greater bodily awareness, increased strength, and more internal locus of control that exercise brings may help to improve the negative attitudes toward the body and alleviate some of the avoidance of sexual activity that often follows physical or sexual trauma.

Role Conflicts and Relationship Concerns. Exercise cannot be expected to solve role conflicts, reduce role overload, or "cure" difficult relationships, but it does help to manage the stress these problems cause. Women with heavy family or work role demands or community commitments often protest that they cannot take time from their busy schedules to engage in regular exercise. They can sometimes be persuaded to make time by telling them that they cannot care for others effectively if they are fatigued, depressed, or physically ill. Exercise, of course, improves mood and energy levels and decreases the risk of many illnesses. Exercise time is more than a temporary escape from stressful routines; while walking, bicycling, or using work-out machines, women can let their minds wander to reflections on their life situations and how they might be altered and improved. Because women with children at home are least likely to exercise (Marcus et al., 1994; Verhoef et al., 1992), therapists might suggest that the women invite their children to join them for a walk, bike ride, or roller skating. Exercise might seem more worthwhile if it can be combined with family fun and quality time for talking, and, of course, children need exercise, too. Partners who feel that they are drifting apart are often advised to take up a new hobby or activity together. Therapists can suggest activities that will also provide physical exercise, such as ballroom or swing dancing lessons, yoga classes, or joining a softball team or bowling league. The improved mood and energy levels may be almost as helpful as spending time together to partners who are attempting to repair relationships.

CONCLUSION

Can exercise contribute to the goals of feminist therapy? We believe that the answer is a resounding "yes." However, encouraging sedentary women to take up a sport or maintain an exercise routine will never be easy; the barriers to exercise are high for many women, and feminist therapists must be creative in supporting and assisting women in moving from contemplating exercise to actually doing it. Is motivation low? Suggest that your client exercise with a friend; women are usually more willing to disappoint themselves than to disappoint their friends. Is the neighborhood an unsafe place to walk or jog? Suggest that your client use an aerobic dance tape at home. Is she uncomfortable being seen in a bathing suit? Suggest that she put swimming on hold for awhile, don a baggy track suit, and start walking. Therapists should be sure to care for the whole person. Remember that exercise helps not only mental health but physical health as well, a message that may be especially important for low income older and ethnic minority women.

Feminist therapy is a revolutionary act (Brown, 1994). So listen to your Aunt Susan, and prescribe some exercise to develop your clients' stamina and resilience. They'll need it to win both the battle for equality and the revolution within (Steinem, 1992).

REFERENCES

Ballou, M., & West, C. (2000). Feminist therapy approaches. In M. Biaggio & M. Hersen (Eds.), *Issues in the psychology of women* (pp. 273-297). New York: Kluwer/Plenum.

Bart, P. B., & O'Brien, P. H. (1985). *Stopping rape: Successful survival strategies.* New York: Pergamon.

Bassey, E. J. (2000). The benefits of exercise for the health of older people. *Reviews in Clinical Gerontology, 10,* 17-31.

Bazargan, M. (1996). Self-reported sleep disturbance among African American elderly: The effects of depression, health status, exercise, and social support. *International Journal of Aging and Human Development, 42,* 143-160.

Berger, B. G., & Owen, D. R. (1983). Mood alteration with swimming: Swimmers really do "feel better." *Psychosomatic Medicine, 45,* 425-433.

Berger, B. G., & Owen, D. R. (1992). Mood alteration with yoga and swimming: Aerobic exercise may not be necessary. *Perceptual and Motor Skills, 75,* 1331-1343.

Blair, S. N., Powell, K. E., Bazzarre, T. L., Early, J. L., Epstein, L. H., Green L. W., Harris, S. S., Haskell, W. L., King, A. C., Koplan, J., Marcus, B. H., Paffenbarger, R. S., & Yeager, K. K. (1993). Physical inactivity workshop V. *Circulation, 88,* 1402-1405.

Brown, L. S. (1994). *Subversive dialogues: Theory in feminist therapy.* New York: Basic Books.

Choi, P. Y. (1992). The psychological benefits of physical exercise: Implications for women and the menstrual cycle. *Journal of Reproductive and Infant Psychology, 10,* 111-115.

Chrisler, J. C., & Ghiz, L. (1993). Body image issues of older women. *Women & Therapy, 14*(1/2), 67-75.

Doyne, E. J., Chambless, D. L., & Beutler, L. E. (1983). Aerobic exercise as a treatment for depression in women. *Behavior Therapy, 14,* 434-440.

Eby, K. K., Campbell, J. C., Sullivan, C. M., & Davidson, W. S. (1995). Health effects of experiences of sexual violence for women with abusive partners. *Health Care for Women International, 16,* 563-576.

Flannery-Schroeder, E. C., & Chrisler, J. C. (1996). Body esteem, eating attitudes, and gender-role orientation in three age groups of children. *Current Psychology, 15,* 235-248.

Gardner, R. M., Stark, K., Friedman, B. N., & Jackson, N. A. (2000). Predictors of eating disorder scores in children ages 6 through 14: A longitudinal study. *Journal of Psychosomatic Research, 49,* 199-205.

Gilligan, C. (1982). *In a different voice: Psychological theory and women's development.* Cambridge, MA: Harvard University Press.

Hall, R. L. (2000). Sweating it out: The good news and the bad news about women and sport. In J. C. Chrisler, C. Golden, & P. D. Rozee (Eds.), *Lectures on the psychology of women* (2nd ed.) (pp. 48-63). New York: McGraw-Hill.

Hartz, G. W., Wallace, W. L., & Clayton, T. G. (1982). Effect of aerobic conditioning upon mood in clinically depressed men and women: A preliminary investigation. *Perceptual and Motor Skills, 55,* 1217-1218.

Hays, K. F. (1994). Running therapy: Special characteristics and therapeutic issues of concern. *Psychotherapy, 31,* 725-734.

Hays, K. F. (1999). *Working it out: Using exercise in psychotherapy.* Washington, DC: American Psychological Association.

Joiner, T. E., & Tickle, J. J. (1998). Exercise and depressive and anxious symptoms: What is the nature of their interactions? *Journal of Occupational Rehabilitation, 8,* 191-198.

Jordan, J., Kaplan, A. G., Miller, J. B., Stiver, I. P., & Surrey, J. L. (1991). *Women's growth in connection: Writings from the Stone Center.* New York: Guilford.

King, A. C., Blair, S. N., Bild, D. E., Dishman, R. K., Duppert, P. M., Marcus, B. H., Oldridge, N. B., Paffenbarger, R. S., Powell, K. E., & Yeager, K. K. (1992). Determinants of physical activity and interventions in adults. *Medicine and Science in Sports and Exercise, 24* (Suppl. 6), S221-S236.

King, A. C., & Kiernan, M. (1997). Physical activity and women's health: Issues and future directions. In S. J. Gallant, G. P. Keita, & R. Royak-Schaler (Eds.), *Health care and women: Psychological, social, and behavioral influences* (pp. 133-146). Washington, DC: APA Books.

Light, K. A., & Girdler, S. A. (1993). Cardiovascular health and disease in women. In C. A. Niven & D. Carroll (Eds.), *The health psychology of women* (pp. 59-73). Langehorn, PA: Harwood.

Malkin, A. R., Wornian, K., & Chrisler, J. C. (1999). Women and weight: Gendered messages on magazine covers. *Sex Roles, 40,* 647-655.

Marcus, B. H., Dubbert, P. M., King, A. C., & Pinto, B. M. (1995). Physical activity in women: Current status and future directions. In A. L. Stanton & S. J. Gallant (Eds.), *The psychology of women's health: Progress and challenges in research and application* (pp. 349-379). Washington, DC: APA Books.

Marcus, B. H., Pinto, B. M., Simkin, L. R., Audrain, J. E., & Taylor, E. R. (1994). Application of theoretical models of exercise behavior among employed women. *American Journal of Health Promotion, 9,* 49-55.

Mathes, S. (1978). Body image and sex stereotyping. In C. Oglesby (Ed.), *Women and sport: From myth to reality* (pp. 59-73). Philadelphia: Lea & Febiger.

Miller, J. B. (1976). *Toward a new psychology of women.* Boston: Beacon Press.

Minor, M. A., & Brown, J. D. (1993). Exercise maintenance of persons with arthritis after participation in a class experience. *Health Education Quarterly, 20,* 83-95.

Nagy, S., & Frazier, S. (1998). The impact of exercise on locus of control. *Journal of Social Behavior and Personality, 3,* 263-268.

Nelson, M. B. (1998). *Embracing victory: Life lessons in competition and compassion.* New York: William Morrow.

Norvell, N., Martin, D., & Salamon, A. (1991). Psychological and physiological benefits of passive and aerobic exercise in sedentary middle-aged women. *Journal of Nervous and Mental Diseases, 179,* 573-574.

O'Leary, M. R. (1992). Self-presentational processes in exercise and sport. *Journal of Sport and Exercise Psychology, 14*, 339-351.

Pate, R. R., Pratt, M., Blair, S. N., Haskell, W. L., Macera, C. A., Bouchard, C., Buchner, D., Caspersen, C. J., Ettinger, W., Heath, G. W., King, A. C., Kriska, A., Leon, A. S., Marcus, B. H., Morris, J., Paffenbarger, R., Patrick, K., Pollock, M. L., Rippe, J. M., Sallis, J., & Wilmore, J. H. (1995). Physical activity and public health: A recommendation from the Centers for Disease Control and Prevention and the American College of Sports Medicine. *Journal of the American Medical Association, 273*, 402-407.

Pettus, M. (2001). Kudos for me: Self-esteem. In J. J. Robert-McComb (Ed.), *Eating disorders in women and children: Prevention, stress management, and treatment* (pp. 283-290). Boca Raton, FL: CRC Press.

Pierce, E. F., & Pate, D. W. (1994). Mood alterations in older adults following acute exercise. *Perceptual and Motor Skills, 79*, 191-194.

Roades, L. A. (2000). Mental health issues for women. In M. Biaggio & M. Hersen (Eds.), *Issues in the psychology of women* (pp. 251-272). New York: Kluwer/Plenum.

Rodin, J., Silberstein, L., & Striegel-Moore, R. (1985). Women and weight: A normative discontent. *Nebraska Symposium on Motivation*, 267-304.

Rozee, P. D. (2000). Freedom from fear of rape: The missing link in women's freedom. In J. C. Chrisler, C. Golden, & P. D. Rozee (Eds.), *Lectures on the psychology of women* (2nd ed.) (pp. 254-269). New York: McGraw-Hill.

Sage, G. H., & Loudermilk, S. (1979). The female athlete and role conflict. *Research Quarterly, 50*, 88-96.

Saltzberg, E. A., & Chrisler, J. C. (1995). Beauty is the beast: Psychological effects of the pursuit of the perfect female body. In J. Freeman (Ed.), *Women: A feminist perspective* (4th ed.) (pp. 306-315). Mountain View, CA: Mayfield.

Snyder, E. E., & Spreitzer, E. (1973). Family influences and involvement in sports. *Research Quarterly, 44*, 249-255.

Steege, J. F., & Blumenthal. J. A. (1993). The effects of aerobic exercise on premenstrual symptoms in middle-aged women: A preliminary study. *Journal of Psychosomatic Research, 37*, 127-133.

Steinem, G. (1992). *Revolution from within: A book of self-esteem.* Boston: Little, Brown.

Steptoe, A., Kimbell, J., & Basford, P. (1998). Exercise and the experience and appraisal of daily stressors: A naturalistic study. *Journal of Behavioral Medicine, 21*, 363-374.

Stuhlmiller, C. M. (1994). Action-based therapy for PTSD. In M. B. Williams & J. F. Sommer, Jr. (Eds.), *Handbook of post-traumatic therapy* (pp. 386-400). Westport, CT: Greenwood.

Thoren, P., Floras, J. S., Hoffman, P., & Seals, D. R. (1990). Endorphins and exercise: Physiological mechanisms and clinical implications. *Medicine & Science in Sports & Exercise, 20*, 417-428.

Verhoef, M. J., Love, E. J., & Rose, M. S. (1992). Women's social roles and their exercise participation. *Women & Health, 19*(4), 15-29.

Vertinsky, P. (1998). Run, Jane, run: Central tensions in the current debate about enhancing women's health through exercise. *Women & Health, 27*(4), 81-111.

Winborn, M. D., Meyers, A. W., & Mulling, C. (1998). The effects of gender and experience on perceived exertion. *Journal of Sport and Exercise Psychology, 10,* 22-31.

Worell, J., & Remer, P. (1992). *Feminist perspectives in therapy: An empowerment model for women.* New York: Wiley.

Latinas:
Exercise and Empowerment
from a Feminist Psychodynamic Perspective

Melba J. T. Vasquez

SUMMARY. Exercise has been identified as an effective intervention to increase well being, and to decrease depression, anxiety and other mental illnesses and disorders (Hayes, 1999). This paper is designed to identify exercise as an important intervention which is conceptually congruent from a feminist psychodynamic perspective. Although this author works from an eclectic approach, and believes it is helpful to conceptualize from a variety of perspectives for various disorders, and for various individuals, the focus of this paper will be to consider the use of exercise from a feminist perspective as applied to psychodynamic psychotherapy. Case examples will be provided, especially ones which reflect work with Latina clients. *[Article copies available for a fee from The Haworth Document Delivery Service: 1-800-HAWORTH. E-mail address: <getinfo@haworthpressinc. com> Website: <http://www.HaworthPress.com> © 2002 by The Haworth Press, Inc. All rights reserved.]*

KEYWORDS. Latinas, psychodynamic therapy, empowerment, exercise

Traditional models of therapy are defined, according to Worell and Remer (1992), as those therapies that put an emphasis on therapist ob-

Address correspondence to: Melba J. T. Vasquez, PhD, ABPP, Vasquez & Associates Mental Health Services, 2901 Bee Cave Road, Box N, Austin, TX 78746.

[Haworth co-indexing entry note]: "Latinas: Exercise and Empowerment from a Feminist Psychodynamic Perspective." Vasquez, Melba J. T. Co-published simultaneously in *Women & Therapy* (The Haworth Press, Inc.) Vol. 25, No. 2, 2002, pp. 23-38; and: *Exercise and Sport in Feminist Therapy: Constructing Modalities and Assessing Outcomes* (ed: Ruth L. Hall, and Carole A. Oglesby) The Haworth Press, Inc., 2002, pp. 23-38. Single or multiple copies of this article are available for a fee from The Haworth Document Delivery Service [1-800-HAWORTH, 9:00 a.m. - 5:00 p.m. (EST). E-mail address: getinfo@haworthpressinc.com].

23

jectivity, analytical thinking, therapist expertness and control of procedures, emotional distance from clients, and intrapsychic dynamics. Worell and Remer (1992) further contend that traditional therapies, such as psychodynamic therapy, involve gender-biased stereotyping and diagnostic labeling, androcentric interpretations, and intrapsychic assumptions. Feminist therapy is a philosophy and feminist therapists use a wide range of theoretical orientations. Although this therapist uses an eclectic approach to therapy with a variety of clients, a feminist transformation of the psychodynamic perspective will be discussed as integrated with the use of exercise as an intervention with Latina clients in particular.

Worell and Remer (1992) suggest that a feminist transformation of a theory should be examined and analyzed according to several criteria. Those criteria indicate that the theories should: be gender free; be flexible in acceptance of life styles and not be heterosexist or ethnocentric; include consideration of environmental experiences and not pathologize; include the lifelong nature of development; assume that the personal is political; strive for and value an egalitarian relationship between therapist and client/patient; and value female value systems and perspectives. To elaborate further, first, the theory should be gender free since, for the most part, women and men are similar in make-up and differences are due to socialization. Second, the theory should be flexible, incorporate a wide range of healthy lifestyles as acceptable, and should not be heterosexist nor ethnocentric. Third, a feminist transformation takes into account that a person's functioning is the result of interactions between individual and environmental experiences. The therapist's conceptualization should not pathologize the individual. Fourth, rather than assume that current patterns of behavior were determined and fixed at an early stage, and are unlikely to change, a therapist should consider development as a lifelong process. Fifth, feminist therapy principles assume that the personal is political and that each individual is limited by sex-role stereotyping, institutionalized sexism, and oppression. Again, the external environment must be considered the main source of client's problems. Sixth, an egalitarian relationship between therapist and client is another basic principle which influences the collaborative process in therapy. The client is considered to be an expert on herself, and the therapist strives to balance the power and affirm the woman client. Last, valuing the female perspective and female value systems through assisting clients to identify the devalued aspects of their socialized selves and focusing on strengths and resilience is another basic principle in feminist approaches to psychotherapy.

While some aspects of psychodynamic therapy are thus incongruent with a feminist approach, many other aspects are useful. For example, helping a client to form a relationship between the conscious and unconscious is a very helpful strategy in working with women. That is, increasing her awareness via a variety of strategies (trusting the dreams, fantasies and other unconscious products of the client as well as her interpretations of her unconscious processes) is a way to affirm the client and to increase her power by increasing self awareness. Identifying strategies described as "defense mechanisms," but redefining them as "coping strategies" reflects a positive feminist framework. Redefining can help a client have compassion for the development of strategies which may have been useful at one time but which may not be helpful currently. A Latina client who learned to withdraw into silence in the context of her family, because being outspoken was seen as a sign of disrespect and elicited punishment, may have a tendency to be hard on herself in the context of interactions which require verbal discussion, but which are intimidating. This client was critical of herself because of her difficulty in speaking up in class. Helping her understand the unconscious functionality of this "automatic coping" reaction to an "unsafe" context can help engender self compassion, even as she works to change her behavior into more assertive verbal expressions.

Furthermore, a shift from a focus on the individual to a focus on environmental effects on the individual, including exploration of the inner world, is a subtle but significant shift. Helping the Latina client described above understand how a seminar consisting mostly of a White professor and white students may be experienced as "unsafe," given previous experiences of discrimination and her experiences in her own family, can help her understand the impact of her environment, both past and present. She alone is not to blame for feeling intimidated; those feelings are not reflective of individual inadequacy of character, but are natural reactions to environmental experiences with discrimination, combined with the learned role in her family of origin. The actual degree of a lack of safety in her current situation is one to be assessed through risk taking.

Client acceptance is defined by many (Worell & Remer, 1992) as the sine qua non of any psychotherapy. Indeed, client acceptance is important to any therapy and is especially important from a feminist approach. Clients are not pathologized for thinking, feeling, and behaving in ways that are congruent with living in their perception of an oppressive society (Worell & Remer, 1992). This acceptance is an initial step in helping the client develop skills and behaviors as part of her empowerment in living as effectively as possible in the challenging society which may be oppressive at times.

In addition, the feminist focus on empowerment is a feminist therapy goal that is the result of increased awareness not only of one's conscious and unconscious but also with an increased awareness of the effects of the environment on the individual. Unlike most traditional psychotherapies, a feminist approach may involve supporting strategies which increase empowerment.

EXERCISE AS A PSYCHOTHERAPEUTIC INTERVENTION

The intervention of exercise as a strategy in psychotherapy can help increase a client's feeling of effectiveness in her life. Recently, research has more clearly supported the use of exercise in increasing one's health and mental health (Hays, 1999). Hays (1999) reviewed a wide range of studies which illustrated the psychological benefits of exercise with such disorders as the following: depression; anxiety; stress management, self-esteem, and mastery; weight loss and gain; substance abuse recovery; chronic mental illness; trauma survivor empowerment; and recovery from medical illness. The research which follows illustrates some these findings.

Depression and the Use of Exercise

One recent study (Blumenthal, Babyak, Moore, Craighead, Herman, Khatri, Waugh, Napolitano, Forman, Applebaum, Doraiswamy, & Krisna, 1999) found that exercise worked at least as well as Zoloft in reducing or eliminating symptoms for patients who had major depression, but were not suicidal or psychotic. Patients who exercised, both men and women, who were at least 50 years old and older, showed greater improvement than those who just took antidepressants and those who took medication and exercised. Furthermore, exercise seemed to be more effective in keeping symptoms from returning after the depression lifted. Blumenthal et al. (1999), who conducted the research, indicated that approximately 60 percent of the exercisers (brisk walking, stationary bike riding or jogging for 30 minutes, three times a week), 66 percent of the medication group, and 69 percent of the combination group had vastly improved or had no symptoms after four months. Ten months later, the researchers found that exercisers who had been in remission after four months were far less likely to see their depression return after

10 months, compared with people taking the medication or a combination therapy. Eight percent of exercisers saw symptoms come back, compared with 38 percent of those patients taking medication and 31 percent in the combination group. Although the findings may not apply to all depression patients, and although group dynamics may have played a role in alleviating depression, this study indicates that exercise may contribute significantly to relieving depressive symptoms. A review of over 80 studies indicates that the most effective antidepressant occurred when exercise and psychotherapy were combined (Hays, 1999). The magnitude of change, however, with exercise alone is significant, and for some individuals, exercise is just as effective as a variety of medical, individual and group psychotherapies (Klein, Greist, Gurmam, Neimeyer, Lesser, Bushnell, & Smith, 1985).

Although mechanisms of effect relating to exercise and depression are uncertain, several hypotheses have been explored. Exercise appears to provide increased self-efficacy. That is, when people begin to change their bodies and look better, they have a greater sense of control. The helplessness that goes along with depression decreases. The sense of mastery may be especially important for women of color, since the person is able to do something they were unable to do before. We may also create more body awareness when we exercise, and that sense of body compared to the numb state during depression can help one feel better. Increase in endorphins (hormones that produce natural feelings of well-being while reducing pain), hypothesized to be a result of aerobic exercise, may also play a role in improving mood. In addition, exercise can help bring the body back into homeostasis once it has responded to the "fight or flight" response to stressful situations, experiences and events. It has also been hypothesized that exercise may help the regulation of neurotransmitters, affecting both mood and ability to cope.

Women experience twice as much depression as men, due to social, economic, biological and emotional factors (McGrath, Keita, Strickland & Russo, 1990). Exercise may serve as a particularly empowering intervention, as perceived mastery is one of the outcomes of exercise for most people. Latina women in particular may benefit from a sense of mastery and action, yet Latinas do not exercise as much as other women (Delgado, 1997). Delgado (1997) suggests that exercise is a must in the overall health of Latinas, and provides a variety of suggestions on how to integrate exercise into one's schedule.

There are indications that the benefits of exercise are almost immediate. Exercise has recently been identified as a primary strategy to maintain good health, and reduce risk of various physical illnesses. Federal guidelines suggest that people should, at the least, walk briskly or use an equivalent amount of energy in some other activity 30 minutes a day on most days, that is, four or five days a week (U. S. Department of Health and Human Services, 1990).

USE OF EXERCISE FROM A PSYCHODYNAMIC PERSPECTIVE

Hays (1999) reported that in the 1960s, sports psychologists approached the field from a personological perspective rooted in psychodynamic theory. An indepth exploration of the meaning of sport/exercise can include the notion that exercise provides an adaptive response to losses that affect self-esteem and produce intrapsychic pain (Sachs, 1981). Although Sachs focused on running, this author believes that any aerobic exercise/sport (walking, bicycling, swimming, dancing, various aerobic gym machines, etc.) can provide benefits described here. From a psychodynamic perspective, a client may be encouraged to free associate thoughts, dreams, fantasies during exercise, to use for material in psychotherapy. For many clients, exercise can be a form of meditation and/or opportunity to allow images and thoughts and feelings to surface and increase awareness and insights. Clients may act out their issues in various ways through exercise. Exercise can be helpful in the exploration of adaptive and maladaptive aspects of coping strategies, transference, countertransference and resistance. For example, a client's resistance to exercise must be addressed as it may be conceptualized as an unconscious barrier. As such, resistance can be explored.

One Latina client, in her late twenties, suffered from depression and grief from her mother's early death caused by a progressive neurological disorder four years earlier. The client, a bright young professional with a master's degree, reported in therapy that she wished to eat more healthily, return to exercise (which she had done consistently for several months but had discontinued prior to coming into therapy), initiate friendships outside of work, and other self care activities. Yet, she found herself "unable" to do so week after week. With therapy, she was able to explore her feelings and thoughts in a more in depth way. She shared the horrors of watching her relatively young mother waste away. She and her sister alternated in caring for their dying mother on evenings and weekends. Care-taking included changing her mother's diapers, feeding her, providing medications, moving her in bed to avoid bed sores, and so on. Her parents were divorced and she and her sister were expected to be her caretakers until her mother was placed in a nursing home shortly before her death. The client wept with anger and frustration stating that she was tired of taking care of others, of struggling, and wanted good things to come to her without any effort on her part! This bright young Latina who had earned a master's degree in a difficult area of study (which indicated persistence and tenacity) was exhausted, still traumatized and suffering from grief, and was subconsciously resisting taking care of herself. This subconscious wish, born of anger, frustration and the unfairness of loss, especially of a mother who herself had been very warm and care-taking, was serving as a barrier for her ability to empower herself to take action. In addition, some transference with the therapist consisted of a wish that the therapist take the role of caretaker, and the frustration that that wish was not gratified contributed to the resistance to take action herself. I will illustrate later in the article how reintroducing exercise as a stress management tool aided her.

STRESSORS AND THE USE OF EXERCISE WITH LATINAS

Hispanics as a group lag in many areas of health. Diabetes, AIDS, obesity and depression are major health problems for Latinas, according to the National Women's Health Information Center (2001). According to Gullo (2000), Dr. Jane Delgado, President of the National Coalition of Hispanic Health and Human Services Organization, suggests that there is variance among subgroups of the culture that require more study: 11 percent of all Hispanics in the United States are Puerto Ricans, 63 percent are Mexican Americans, 4 percent are Cubans, and 22 percent are South and Central Americans. These cultural groups differ in significant ways, and such differences can affect therapy approaches including exercise. Furthermore, Delgado stated that Hispanics with lower incomes are also in poorer health.

On the other hand, there is much evidence of resilience among these groups. Hispanics live longer than whites and Hispanic women have lower rates of breast cancer (but more cervical cancer) than non-Hispanic women (Delgado, 1997). The fast-growing Hispanic population has had an historically low rate of welfare dependency, a high rate of participation in the labor force, good life expectancy rates, and a high percentage of healthy babies. In fact, according to the Texas Department of Health's Bureau of Vital Statistics (*Austin American Statesman*, December 11, 1996, p. B4), Hispanic baby girls born in 1995 will have the highest life expectancy of any racial or gender groups as they are expected to live an average 80.3 years. Because extended families provide emotional support, Hispanic women are less likely to live alone, are less likely to be smokers or drinkers, may have a better diet, and their infant mortality rate is lower than other groups.

Despite these aspects of resiliency, Latina women, like many women of color, experience oppressive and biased responses on a regular basis in the workplace and in other settings. Exercise is one strategy which not only helps to manage the effects of such stress and the resulting symptoms of depression, anxiety, and post traumatic stress disorder, but can also help promote confidence, strength and promote creative thought processes in handling and implementing responses to such stresses.

One potential stressor for women in general, and Latinas in particular, includes the demands of caregiving (Delgado, 1997; Dreyfuss, 2000). The lack of time and feelings of weariness can be powerful obstacles to exercise. Nurturing others could potentially block a path to the nurturer's own better health. We are just beginning to understand how these caregiving acts for children and for other relatives can be quite burdensome and can reduce time for self care.

Dreyfuss (2000) reported the results of a telephone-based outreach, in which counselors encouraged women caregivers to be more active (Bull, Eyler, King & Brownson, 2001). The program also gave them advice on how being more active can be successful. Women who benefited from the physical activity were women ages 50 and older who were caring for a relative with dementia. The women were able to increase their activity levels, and even get better sleep. Care-giving will be a responsibility for more people as the Baby Boom population ages. Women tend to live longer than men and tend, in the older age groups, to be a caregiver for a spouse. If a telephone intervention can effectively encourage women to increase their activity level, which will also increase emotional well being, encouragement in our therapeutic intervention strategies may have an even greater effect!

Latina women face unique issues. Delgado (1997) who, along with the National Hispanic Women's Health Initiative, published *Salud! A Latina's Guide to Total Health: Body, Mind, and Spirit,* includes exercise as a chapter in the "Living Well" section of her book. She described the fact that Hispanic women are known for placing family needs above their own all their lives, which can serve as a barrier to self care and for exercise in particular.

However, Latina women are becoming more aware that caring for themselves is as important as caring for others. Indeed, self care is one of the most important general interventions for all women, and for Latina women in particular. It is easy for a Latina who is part of a family, for example, to understand that if the health of a woman collapses, the health of the family of which she is the center collapses as well.

Not only does exercise help manage depression, stress and anxiety, but it helps us be literally stronger, look better, helps us manage our lives better, have greater energy and vitality, and thus feel happier. It also helps us keep perspectives when unfair, racist, sexist and/or heterosexist, events "trigger" overreactions and/or old, faulty destructive coping or defense reactions. A more positive mindset helps keep negative experiences in perspective. With support from others (family, friends, support groups, therapists) a positive mindset can prevent self blame and negative self attributions, which so often lead to depression and anxiety after those painful events. Understanding the unfair societal oppression is painful, but the effects can be partially ameliorated when one is engaged in healthy self care, and experiencing its benefits.

The following case illustrates the use of exercise to manage various presenting concerns and stressors including depression, anxiety, maladaptive coping patterns, lack of assertiveness, and other challenges. The use of exercise to increase the feelings of confidence, self esteem, increased awareness and personal power were goals for this Latina client in particular, who was in her late thirties when she entered therapy again. She had suffered various losses, abuses and abandonments, and had been a client on and off for a dozen years. Much of her therapy has been insight oriented, although cognitive behavioral interventions were also used; all from a feminist perspective. When she first entered therapy, she was depressed, suicidal, abusing alcohol, and confused about life. She was unhappily married, and angrily and astutely aware of the discrimination and oppression in her life. She suffered from "insidious post traumatic stress disorder," and often became symptomatic when witnessing or experiencing injustice. Yet, she had many strengths. A major intervention was for her to begin to exercise, which typically involved either fast walking or running, and some weight training, three to five times a week. At times, she exercised with others, which was her preference, but she worked on maintaining her schedule regardless of whether friends could join her. She worked to substitute exercise instead of drinking alcohol in order to deal with stress, pain and anxiety of daily living, as well as to manage her destructive reactions when she got "triggered" by unfairness or abuse around her. She first had to become aware of the warning signs both in her environment as well as within herself, which triggered stressful experiences and unhappy emotions. She was bright, and very open to learning more effective communication and coping strategies. She gained various skills and made considerable progress over the years.

The client returned to therapy as a result of several incidents. She was aware of feeling distress as a result of several well publicized racist and discriminatory events in the media, as well as in her life. She called me after she nearly acted out physically with a white racist colleague. An African American colleague of hers was retiring. At the office party, the racist colleague entered the room, said nothing to the departing colleague, partook of the refreshments and left the room. My client followed her colleague out of the room. In her "previous life," my client would have indulged her impulse and may have become verbally or physically abusive to the colleague. Instead, my client made a sarcastic comment, returned to her desk, left early, and went to the gym. She realized that day that she had not been exercising as regularly as she needed to in order to manage her stress, anger, lack of safety and powerlessness, angst and other symptoms. She remembered how during exercise, she could better sort out and plan a healthier reaction to those incidents. Part of her return to short term therapy involved supporting her to rebuild her exercise program!

OTHER EXAMPLES OF EXERCISE AS INTERVENTION

Encouragement of clients to maintain overall health of body, mind and spirit is an important element of a feminist approach to psychodynamic therapy, in which health, fitness and exercise are important strategies. In doing so, we must also encourage clients to be realistic in their exercise goals. Exercise is for the goal of getting "fit." Although regular exercise helps us look better, this is not the same as looking like a fashion model and fitness must be the primary goal of exercise. It is also critical to encourage clients to be patient; often clients are discouraged by previous attempts and "false starts." Clients should be reminded that research on the change process indicates that so called "false starts" are actually part of the process of behavior/habit change. This concept is part of my eclectic approach to psychotherapy. The Latina client who was grieving for her mother, feeling abandoned, and whom I described as resisting returning to exercise, even though she had benefited from it before, had stopped exercising partly because she had not lost weight after several months of consistent exercise. She worked to accept "fitness" as a goal, rather than weight loss. Also, she was very self critical about stopping and having to start over until we reconceptualized her efforts as an over-all process of incorporating exercise as a regular lifestyle event, compa-rable to brushing one's teeth. Behavior change and new habits often require beginning again after a "relapse." In addition, it is important to be forgiving of oneself when one gets off the exercise plan, and this was a very important goal in general for this client.

Confidence building is an important goal for many Latinas. Regard-less of how supportive are the families of origin, the oppression in soci-ety resulting from racism, sexism, heterosexism and classism can affect one's sense of self. Confidence building in therapy takes various forms, depending on the needs of the client. Increased awareness of oneself and the effects of the environment on oneself can involve, for example, helping clients to see that, given the oppression in society, goals can of-ten be thwarted by institutional "isms," biased supervisors and the like. The research conducted by Dovidio and Gaertner (1996, 2000), for ex-ample, illustrates that discrimination in various aspects of the selection process in employment and school admissions is still very prevalent, subconscious, and easily rationalized by perpetrators. These insights can be very helpful to clients. In addition, clients benefit from examin-ing their productive and destructive responses to those unfortunate events.

Clients can develop psychological and physical strengths and resil-ience through the development of confidence. Often, clients develop confidence by taking action and accomplishing small goals on a daily basis. Exercise can be one of those goals. I encourage clients to stay ac-tive, and to "lean into" unresolved and/or bothersome issues when pos-sible. In other words, the avoidance of aversive tasks/issues can lead to anxiety and/or depression. Exercise is one activity over which most women can have control. Moreover, exercise can generate the energy to tackle difficult issues/activities in ones life. One Latina client, who was "stuck" in her inability to make progress on her dissertation, had experi-enced a serious drop in her confidence and ability to produce the work she needed to in order to obtain her PhD. She suffered from moderate symptoms of obsessive compulsive disorder (OCD), including nega-tive, obsessive thoughts. She began exercise (swimming and bicycling) as part of her goal of generating more energy, and managing the anxiety underlying her OCD. During exercise, she both free associated her fears and anxieties (which led to discovery in therapy of sources of fears) as well as visualized herself working at her computer, or in the library to make progress on her dissertation, which required "leaning into her anxiety." The client was able to then act on the visualization and make progress.

Clients are encouraged to begin where they can, and to increase exercise to a minimum of three times a week, with five or six times a week an optimal goal for those wishing to manage depression and anxiety symptoms in particular. Exercise can be diverse, or a client may choose to engage in a favorite one. Aerobic activity is important for stress management, as it re-regulates the central nervous system, and brings the body back into homeostasis. Increased awareness can be helpful for clients regarding the benefits of bringing the body back to normal after the body engages in the "fight or flight" reaction in response to stress (a daily occurrence for most of us). Exercise literally makes us feel better because of the endorphins, hormones that produce natural feelings of well being while reducing pain. It also increases cardiovascular efficiency, makes our lungs function better which together carries the nutrients in our blood throughout our bodies and take away the wastes and toxins.

From my eclectic model of psychotherapy, I remind clients that habit development and formation takes approximately 8-12 weeks. If one gets "out of the habit" of exercise as a life style, one can reestablish it. Encouraging clients to gain support from those around her is also important. Exercising with one's partner and/or friends can help enhance the experience and commitment; clients should also be encouraged to exercise whether others can join her or not. One Latina client, in her mid fifties, who experienced a major trauma–the murder of her daughter–benefited from the fact her friends ensured that she walked almost daily for months and months, based on my suggestion that it might be helpful. The physiological and psychological benefits of the exercise as well as the support from friends helped mediate the intensity of the grief. What's more, her friends became "addicted" to the process of exercise, and I still see several of them on the hike and bike trail where I run on a regular basis.

Developing and cultivating a happy and peaceful attitude is also part of the strategies associated with promotion of overall health. It is helpful to encourage clients to work on awareness about issues/events/people and situations which are worrisome. Latinas can work with and utilize Burns' (1999) *Feeling Good* exercises, developed to promote positive and realistic belief systems, as distinct from beliefs based on fears, and negative assumptions. What's more, often clients can work on their concerns while exercising. I encourage clients to assume the best about a situation (even when they are correctly perceiving bias or unfair treatment), and to practice/visualize behaving in a difficult situation with integrity and dignity. This means acting clearly, assertively, and dropping out destructive reactions. One Latina single mother in her forties, worried about her two teenage children, both of whom were "acting out" in various ways, worried constantly about them, and her interactions with them. She also worried about whether they were treated fairly by others (their father, from whom she was divorced, his new partner, the school principal, their teachers and their friends). We developed a process by which she allowed herself to "check in" with herself about her feelings and thoughts about her teenagers while exercising, deciding on any action to be taken, with them or with others. If any action was to be taken, she was to assume the best about the outcome. She was also to assume the best about her son and daughter in any given situation. She even learned to be aware of whether historical issues from her own experience were being triggered by her teenager's experiences, which she could be, in part, projecting onto her teenagers' situations.

INEFFECTIVE INTERVENTIONS

There are many reasons why people do not exercise. Some do not like competition; others believe that exercise is inspired by vanity and self-indulgence. Other common excuses include no time, too tired, no place, no one to do it with, wrong clothes, too expensive, too boring (Delgado, 1997). Although exercise can serve as an "antidepressant," some clients are too depressed to get the activity cycle going. Psychotherapy and/or medication may be a critical part of the initial intervention. Exercise can then increase and sustain benefits.

Many Latinas who work in highly active service activities (cleaning homes/hotel rooms, outdoor construction or landscaping) may not find exercise at the beginning or end of the day appealing. Other strategies involving self care may be helpful. In addition, a discussion of aerobic and anaerobic exercise may be relevant. That is, flexibility, endurance and strength may be gained through their work activities, but the cardiovascular benefits from aerobic exercise, after 30 minutes of sustained exercise with increased heartbeat, may not be.

It is very important, when encouraging clients, especially Latinas, that we not evoke shame and feelings of failure. That fragile balance of challenge and support is critical for clients of color who have often been shamed and made to feel unworthy. One forty-five year old Latina, for example, whose physical illness was unclear and possibly fibromyalgia or some kind of chronic fatigue syndrome, was depressed, angry, could not relate to doctors, and had not been able to tolerate any medications including various antidepressants. I thought she might be prime for exercise, and we worked hard to develop a very light, self-determined strategy to attempt to exercise. However, when I challenged her on some attitudes toward others, she took a break from therapy, and expressed how demanding I was in expecting her to do too much. My failure to convey my concerns in a more accepting way, after challenging her to engage in exercise for someone for whom exercise was such a challenge, went "over the edge" for her.

ETHICAL CONSIDERATIONS

Psychologists and psychotherapists exercise more than the average citizen, and approximately 50% to 75% of therapists report regular physical exercise as part of their self care (Coster & Schwebel, 1997; Hays, 1999; Mahoney, 1997). Exercising, by the psychotherapist, models healthy self care behavior, and demonstrates that we implement what we recommend ourselves. The risk in exercising in small communities is that we will run into clients or former clients in gyms, running trails, bicycle trails, swimming pools, and other exercise locations. It is generally recommended to process clients' feelings in therapy ahead of time, if we know that seeing them will be probable, or after the fact upon occurrence. Confidentiality issues should be discussed, as well as clients' preference to acknowledge each others' presence.

Psychodynamic therapists tend to hold to more stringent boundaries than those from other theoretical orientations (Pope & Vasquez, 1998). The risk of voluntarily spending any time with the client outside of the therapeutic situation is the introduction of a dual relationship, which is problematic because the needs of the psychotherapist often get in the way of the therapy, so boundaries typically involve avoiding such contact.

Hays (1999) conducted a survey designed to examine the function of exercise in the lives of mental health practitioners. One of the questions involved the use of exercise with clients during therapy. The vast majority indicated that they have not and would not, primarily because of interpersonal boundaries, potential liability and malpractice issues, and the concern about promoting a dependent relationship which might inhibit clients' risk taking in finding new exercise partners. However, some therapists working in inpatient settings, as well as with structured outpatient clients, did report doing so. Hays suggested that those considering doing so need to examine questions of boundaries, intimacy, competition, dual role relationships, aggression, dependency, eroticization, and power as well as potential issues of legal liability and confidentiality. For the psychodynamic therapist, issues of transference and countertransference need especially careful attention. Hays further identifies several other ethical issues, including the importance of acquiring specific knowledge of the physiological and social bases of exercise and sport as well as knowledge of the applied sport psychology literature.

CONCLUSION

The impact of exercise on mental health is undeniably positive, and well supported in the literature. It can be incorporated in any number of theoretical approaches, including a psychodynamic approach. An approach in therapy which addresses the overall health of clients, especially women, is important in the empowerment process of those who experience insidious and pervasive oppression in their lives. Therapy can be a painful and difficult process, and interventions which provide clients with tools and skills to gain effectiveness, power and control in their lives are important. Teaching Latinas, especially, to value themselves, is part of the approach and consequence of promoting exercise and physical activity for clients.

REFERENCES

Austin American Statesman, December 11, 1996, "Hispanic girls' life expectancy longest," p. B4-B5.

Blumenthal, J. A., Babyak, M. A., Moore, K. A., Craighead, W. E., Herman, S., Khatri, P., Waugh, R., Napolitano, M. A., Forman, L. M., Applebaum, M., Doraiswamy, P. M., & Krishnan, K. R. (1999). Effects of exercise training on older patients with major depression. *Archive of Internal Medicine, 159,* 2349-2356.

Bull, F. C., Eyler, A. A., King A. C., & Brownson, R. C. (2001). Stage of readiness to exercise in ethnically diverse women: A U. S. survey. *Medical Science in Sports Exercise, 33,* 1147-1156.

Burns, D. D. (1999, revised). *Feeling Good: The New Mood Therapy.* New York: Penguin Books.

Coster, J. S. & Schwebel, M. (1997). Well-functioning in professional psychologists. *Professional Psychology: Research & Practice, 28,* 5-13.

Delgado, J. L. (1997). *Salud! A Latina's Guide to Total Health–Body, Mind, and Spirit.* New York: Harper Collins.

Dovidio, J. F. (2001, January). Why can't we get along? Interpersonal Biases and Interracial Distrust. Presented at the National Multicultural Conference and Summit II, Santa Barbara, CA.

Dovidio, J. F. & Gaertner, S. L. (1996). Affirmative action, unintentional racial biases, and intergroup relations. *Journal of Social Issues, 52*, pp. 51-76.

Dovidio, J. F. & Gaertner, S. L. (2000). Aversive racism and selection decisions: 1989 and 1999. *Psychological Science, 11*(4), 315-319.

Dreyfuss, I. (2000, August 1). *Caregiving: An obstacle to exercise.* Associated Press.

Gullo, K. (2000, February 24). *Study Looks at Health of Hispanics.* Associated Press.

Hays, K. L. (1999). *Working it out: Using exercise in psychotherapy.* Washington, DC: American Psychological Association.

Klein, M. H., Greist, J. H., Gurman, A. S., Neimeyer, R. A., Lesser, D. P., Bushnell, N. J. & Smith, R. E. (1985). A comparative outcome study of group psychotherapy vs. exercise treatments for depression. *International Journal of Mental Health, 13*, 148-177.

Mahoney, M. J. (1997). Psychotherapists' personal problems and self-care patterns. *Professional Psychology: Research & Practice, 28*, 14-16.

McGrath, E., Keita, G. P., Srickland, B. R. & Russo, N. F. (1990). *Women and Depression.* Washington, DC: American Psychological Association.

McKeown, L. A. (2000, June 13). For Women, a Walk a Day Keeps Stroke Away: Exercise May Reverse Risks Piled Up by Years of Sedentary Behavior.

National Women's Health Information Center, Office on Women's Health, U.S. Department of Health and Human Services (2001). Latina Women's Health. http://www.4woman.gov/faq/latina.htm.

Ondash, E. (2000, September 20). *Move it or lose it: Depression, that is.* Health Scout Reporter.

Pope, K. S. & Vasquez, M. J. T. (1998, 2nd ed.). *Ethics in Psychotherapy and Counseling: A Practical Guide.* San Francisco: Jossey-Bass.

Sachs, M. L. (1981). Running addiction. In M. H. Sacks & M. L. Sachs (Eds.). *Psychology of running.* Champagn, IL: Human Kinetics. pp. 116-126.

U.S. Department of Health and Human Services/U.S. Department of Agriculture (1990). *Dietary Guidelines for Americans,* Washington, DC.

Worell, J. & Remer, P. (1992). *Feminist perspectives in therapy: An empowerment model for women.* New York: John Wiley & Sons.

Exercise and Movement
as an Adjunct to Group Therapy
for Women with Chronic Mental Illness

Linda Naylor Dench

SUMMARY. A variety of techniques to promote movement and exercise were used as an adjunct to therapy in an ongoing support group for women with severe and chronic mental health problems. Three women and a therapist had met weekly for 16 weeks at the time of this writing. A short case history of each of the women including a psychiatric assessment, notes on medication regimen, symptomatology, psychosocial history and immediate challenges is presented. Life styles by self-report ranged from sedentary to moderately active. Techniques to "jump start" greater mobility and exercise included: (a) completion of partner interviews on sport, exercise, and movement, (b) construction of a genogram rating the activity level and sport/movement/exercise history of family members, (c) games involving throwing and general movement, and (d) individual walk-talk therapy sessions. As an adjunct to therapy, these techniques followed other expressive therapeutic techniques such as art therapy, sandtray, and dream work. Therapeutic board games and client-centered therapy were also part of the milieu. Most of the techniques to facilitate movement and exercise took place during the last six weeks of the support group. Attitudes toward these techniques and results varied among the participants. *[Article copies available for a fee from The Haworth Document Delivery Service: 1-800-HAWORTH.*

Linda Naylor Dench is affiliated with Temple University.

Address correspondence to: Linda Naylor Dench, 260 Tranquil Heights Lane, Emmaus, PA 18049 (E-mail: lndench@aol.com).

[Haworth co-indexing entry note]: "Exercise and Movement as an Adjunct to Group Therapy for Women with Chronic Mental Illness." Dench, Linda Naylor. Co-published simultaneously in *Women & Therapy* (The Haworth Press, Inc.) Vol. 25, No. 2, 2002, pp. 39-55; and: *Exercise and Sport in Feminist Therapy: Constructing Modalities and Assessing Outcomes* (ed: Ruth L. Hall, and Carole A. Oglesby) The Haworth Press, Inc., 2002, pp. 39-55. Single or multiple copies of this article are available for a fee from The Haworth Document Delivery Service [1-800-HAWORTH, 9:00 a.m. - 5:00 p.m. (EST). E-mail address: getinfo@haworthpressinc.com].

39

E-mail address: <getinfo@haworthpressinc.com> Website: <http://www.Haworth Press.com> © 2002 by The Haworth Press, Inc. All rights reserved.]

KEYWORDS. Chronically mentally ill, exercise, women, support group

BACKGROUND

Studies of exercise in the population with severe psychiatric disabilities are scarce in psychotherapeutic literature (Hays, 1999; Martinsen, 1987). In part, this may be due to the fact that, until the 1970s and 1980s, the majority of individuals with chronic mental illness were treated on a long-term basis in hospitals (Andreasen, 1994). Following the deinstitutionalization movement of the 1970s and 1980s, as many state psychiatric hospitals were closed, treatment of severe psychiatric disabilities became the responsibility of the community (Andreasen, 1994; McFarland, 1994). Of the state hospitals that remain, psychiatric treatment is often restricted to involuntary patients (Andreasen, 1994; McFarland, 1994).

As pointed out by McFarland (1994), community mental health program services vary, with differences in funding affecting the types of services available to this population. These services tend to be minimal involving basic needs such as diagnosis, medication management, and obtaining food, shelter, and clothing. Even where highly desirable services, such as psychosocial services are included, these tend to be in the area of vocational training and supported employment.

Although research in exercise and health dates back to 1884, little research appeared with exercise as an independent variable until the 1970s (Rejeski & Thompson, 1993). It has been theorized that the concept of mind-body dualism inherent in the traditional biomedical model obscured the more contemporary view, in psychosomatic medicine, behavioral medicine, and health psychology, that there is an interdependence between the body, the mind and the social fabric of the individual (Rejeski & Thompson, 1993). The 1980s were notable for the growth of research exploring the therapeutic value of exercise in the mental health arena (Rejeski & Thompson, 1993). Only recently has research begun to expand to the population with severe and chronic mental illness.

I am a mental health therapist in private practice in Pennsylvania. My academic background includes degrees in physical education and counseling psychology. I am a candidate for a doctoral degree with a specialization in exercise and sport psychology at Temple University. The topic of this paper reflects the current direction of my academic work and therapy practice.

Years of experience as a physical education major, certified aerobics instructor, ballroom dancer and life-long sport enthusiast provided the background for appreciating the personal growth and healing aspects of physical activity. As the former Executive Director of a mental health and drug and alcohol facility, it became apparent in supervising approximately a thousand cases, that the clients who tended to be actively involved in sport, exercise, or movement were also the healthiest. Unfortunately, this portion of the population was in the minority of those seeking subsidized counseling services. The majority of clients presented with poor daily living skills and were often quite sedentary.

Funding of programs for these individuals often precluded innovative techniques; the result of the lack of financial resources was that therapy tended to be short term and rather limited. Over the years, the revolving-door nature of this population became increasingly disconcerting. Budget restraints capped the number of sessions and the type of therapy provided.

The impetus for this paper was a desire to get to the root of severe and chronic mental health problems by providing the most comprehensive clinical treatment possible including physical activity modes. As a clinician in private practice, the restrictions encountered in subsidized community mental health treatment programs were no longer a barrier to treatment. Thus, the opportunity to further knowledge and understanding of the value of exercise and movement as an adjunct to traditional treatment in severe and chronic mental illness presented itself.

Three women clients, presenting with chronic and serious conditions, were slated to begin a comprehensive mental health treatment including psychiatric supervision of supportive counseling. The inclusion of appropriate physical activity was approved and subsequently accepted by the clients. It was theorized that an investigation of the sport, exercise, and movement background of the clients, as well as their current activity level, would provide the most appropriate history from which to construct an adjunctive exercise program. Additionally, since a group experience was a component of each individual's treatment plan, it was postulated that this modality could be utilized to motivate each individual to return to, or embrace, a healthier balance of movement and exercise as a daily living skill. To that end, games, movement, partner interviews, and surveys were utilized as an underpinning for individualized walk-talk therapy session. The experiences I describe here support my belief that the inclusion of therapeutic techniques to facilitate a return to, and perhaps even an enhancement of sport, exercise, and movement in the lives of women with severe and chronic mental illness, is a highly desirable adjunct to traditional group therapy. Within many limitations of this in-the-field case study, I have explored techniques to facilitate exercise and movement in a three person group of adult women with a chronic mental illness of at least five years duration.

GROUP PARTICIPANTS

Three women between the ages of 39 and 48 years, referred to in this paper as "WC," "SN," and "PG," were selected by their psychiatrist for group therapy. All members have a history of psychiatric hospitalization and were followed monthly on an individual outpatient basis for psychiatric care. Two of the women were monitored for possible involuntary admission. All were simultaneously involved in individual counseling with the group therapist. Two of the women are married; one is single. The women who are married have husbands who are employed. One of the married women is employed; the single woman works part time.

A brief case history of each woman including a multiaxial psychiatric assessment, medication regimen, symptomatology, psychosocial history and immediate challenges is discussed. Considerations of pathology in treatment planning and the various therapeutic techniques to facilitate exercise and movement are explored as well.

MENTAL HEALTH BACKGROUND OF PARTICIPANTS

Client One: WC is a 48-year-old, single, Caucasian female who has been diagnosed as follows: disorders were noted on all axes including Schizoaffective Disorder, Borderline Personality Disorder, a history of intense mood swings, impulsive and self-mutilating behavior, menopausal dysphoria, and mild to moderate stressors of various types. Her current GAF score was 65. Her medication regimen includes Zyprexa, Wellbutrin, Prozac, Lithobid, Propranolol, and Valium.

Symptomatically, WC has mood swings including anger and temper, fears going to work, experiences nightmares and sleep disturbance. Concentration is "poor," with a tendency to self-isolate. WC perceives her appetite as "too good." She experiences obsessions and compulsions. She has maintained three and one-half years recovery from both drug and alcohol use with one incidence of relapse several weeks into the group. She has a history of anorexia and self-mutilation.

Both of her parents are deceased. She has one married sister. WC has never been married, though she did live with a man who was an abusive alcoholic for seven years. She has a strong attachment to her three dogs.

At the outset of group, WC worked part time for a dog groomer; however, within a period of eight weeks she lost that job as well as a subsequent one. These losses catapulted her into a more dependent state and her obsessive behavior escalated.

Client Two: SN is a 47-year-old, married, Caucasian, who has been diagnosed as follows: Schizophrenia, Paranoid Type (Axis I), Fibromyalgia (Axis III), and mild to moderate stressors (Axis IV). Her GAF is 65. Currently SN is taking Effexor, Klonopin, Risperdal, Detrol, Zocor, Prilosec Inderal, and DayPro. She is allergic to sulfa products.

Her psychiatric records indicated a history of psychotic episodes with paranoid delusions and depressive symptoms. SN reports an inability to get out of bed and to interact socially. She has fibromyalgia pain syndrome, and is symptomatic for diffuse pain with an achiness around her knees and arms, and tenderness in the neck, low back, knees, and hips. There is a slight limitation of motion to her right shoulder. Her cardiac exam was normal and she has had no pulmonary problem. Her physician noted that she has been "out of shape" and had a "marked weight gain on the medications."

SN reports her life changed dramatically after she married her first husband. She left a secure job, family, and friends to move to California where she endured an unstable and unhappy marriage for ten years before returning home with her two sons. She remarried two years ago, and now also has a stepdaughter.

Stressors in her life include living in an unsafe neighborhood in an apartment with too few rooms for herself, her husband and children to have privacy. There are also social, health, family and financial stressors. SN is unemployed because she experienced the pressure of a vocational rehabilitation position (secretarial-clerical assistant) as overwhelming.

Client Three: PG is a 39-year-old Caucasian female whose diagnostic information is as follows: Major Depressive Disorder with psychotic features and Post Traumatic Stress Disorder (Axis I), Avoidant Personality Disorder (Axis II), and mild to moderate stressors (Axis IV). Her GAF has ranged from 45 to 75 in the past year. Her medication regimen currently is as follows: Klonapin, Effexor, Compazine, Remeron and Topamax.

Symptomatically, PG has suicidal ideation almost daily. She has an intense preoccupation with death. She experiences pervasive feelings of danger, futility, fear, anxiety, and confusion. She also has a history of self-mutilation and was hospitalized approximately one year ago when she attempted suicide in her therapist's office. Her extraordinary anxiety and agitation is evidenced by ringing hand movements and the fact that she is barely able to respond to questions of almost any nature. She presents as being "shut down," and often experiences sleep disturbance. At times she complains of nausea. About a month ago she injured her right wrist, and is currently undergoing chiropractic treatment and orthopedic testing.

PG has no alcohol or other drug history; however, she is an adult child of an alcoholic (ACOA) and is an incest survivor. Her post traumatic stress disorder may have initiated following the death of her brother when she was approximately eight years old. Shortly following that, her father attempted suicide. PG reports incestuous molestation as a young adult by a brother-in-law. At the outset of group, she had just completed a period of intense monitoring following a suicide threat. PG is married with three children. She reports marital difficulty, stress at her current job as a nurses' aide, and an obsession with suicidal ideation.

PATHOLOGY AS A CONSIDERATION IN GROUP TREATMENT PLANNING

Given the relatively severe nature of the psychiatric illness and the medication regimen of the participants, safety was primary. A review of related literature supported the concept of exercise as a therapeutic modality although most of the literature focuses on the general population and a relative paucity exists in the area of exercise with chronic patients. The growing body of literature on the efficacy of exercise and mental health in general populations includes studies by Brewer and Petrie (1996), Brown (1987), Buffone (1997), Griest (1987), Hays (1999), Harris (1987), Kostrubala (1997), Martinsen (1987), Sachs (1997), Sime (1987), and Summers and Wolstat (1997). Some of this research focuses on the incidence of psychopathology within the athletic population such as eating disorders, substance-related disorders, the relationship between psychological variables and athletic injury, adjustment reactions, staleness, anxiety reactions and personality disorders (Brewer & Petrie, 1996). Much has also been written on both the positive (healthy habits) and negative aspects of running addiction (Sachs, 1997).

Other research reviewed, with exercise as an independent variable, and improvement in mental health functioning as a dependent variable, targeted psychiatric outpatients (Brown, 1987; Hays, 1999), new mental health clinic patients with depression (Griest, 1987), depression in a mental health clinic of a large university (Harris, 1987), outpatient psychotherapy (Hays, 1999), psychiatric outpatients in group therapy (Kostrubala, 1997), the inpatient population of a psychiatric clinic (Martinsen, 1987), and a selected outpatient case study (Sime, 1987).

Although this research portends the efficacy of exercise as an adjunct to therapy, the challenge remains, nevertheless, for the practitioner to determine the degree to which the characteristics of the target population or case study match her individual client. With safety as the first concern, and with many factors unknown, each of the women described here was viewed as unique with regard to their personal, psychiatric and medical history, sport, exercise and movement history, current symptomatology, and psychological strength and weaknesses. Yet to be discovered was the exact pathway to lead them to their full potential in sport, exercise, movement, and overall health.

One of the important unknowns to be considered was the interactive effect of psychotropic drugs on exercise (Martinsen, 1987). In the present study, a decision was made at the outset to proceed slowly and with great caution. Medical approval was sought from the supervising psychiatrist. Each activity was introduced as a separate building block, and the results assessed before another was added. Accordingly, the comfort level of the participants was factored into the degree of concentration in the sport, movement, exercise area in implementing the techniques that follow.

PARTNER INTERVIEW
ON SPORT, EXERCISE AND MOVEMENT

Each client was asked to interview one of the other group members. There were seven questions on the first interview survey (Table 1): two pertained to sport history; two pertained to preferences in movement and exercise; one was directed to body weight; one required the participants to recall a time in her life when she experienced the greatest sense of being fit; and one explored current exercise practice, desire to exercise daily, and obstacles, if any, to that goal. Respondents were asked to

TABLE 1. Responses to Sport/Exercise/Movement Partner Interview

Questions	Responses by WC	Responses by SN
1. Favorite type of movement.	Walking.	Swing, jitterbug, free-style, slow-dancing, jazz, tap, ballet.
2. List any sports you have ever played.	Football, basketball, baseball, volleyball, badminton, bowling, cross-country, sailing, swimming, canoeing, white water rafting.	Basketball, football, softball, field hockey, bowling, tennis, skiing, skating, volleyball, badminton.
3. List any teams you have ever been on.	Basketball, volleyball in college and high school.	Junior high school: basketball, field hockey. Adult: bowling.
4. Favorite type of exercise?	Walking, treadmill.	Dancing.
5. At what point in your life did you feel the best physically?	1983. Walked my whippet about 10 miles/day. Swam 12 laps. Lifted weights.	1975-1979 (ages 20-25)
6. Ideal weight? How many pounds would you have to gain or lose?	100 pounds. I would have to lose 25 pounds.	Preferred not to say. I would have to lose 68 pounds.
7. Would you like to exercise every day? Do you? If not, what stops you?	Yes. No. Not belonging to the gym any more.	Yes. No. Lack of energy and motivation.

answer each question with the following key: "Never," "Rarely," "Sometimes," "Often," "Always." The survey yielded new information that was pertinent to formulating treatment goals. Client WC stated that she believed that she had been addicted to exercise at the time of her highest level of physical functioning. This period was punctuated by acting out through self-mutilation. She further reported that after walking her dog about ten miles and swimming twelve laps in the pool, that she exercised until she went to bed. SN wistfully confided that "if I thought my heart and lungs could stand it, I would enjoy taking a tap class." GP is not included in this interviewing due to her absence because of a psychiatric crisis during that group session.

Following this exercise, participants were informed that they could elect to do walk-talk therapy during their individual sessions. SN has chosen two such sessions to date while WC has had one such session.

PARTNER INTERVIEW 2
ON SPORT, EXERCISE AND MOVEMENT

The following week, Survey 2 (Table 2) was given for the purpose of gathering information on attitudes and practices with regard to exercise and movement.

Questions 1 and 2 were used as much to plant seeds for lifestyle change as to elicit information. Question 3 sought information on which to potentially build future activities. Questions 4 and 5 were considered key questions to access each individual's practice with regard to exercising and the results thereof. Question 6 was used to determine how receptive participants were at this point for greater focus on exercise.

SPORT/EXERCISE/MOVEMENT GENOGRAM
AS AN ASSESSMENT OF FAMILIAL INFLUENCE

The following week information was obtained on how family of origin potentially influenced core attitudes and beliefs regarding sport, ex-

TABLE 2. Responses to Sport/Exercise/Movement Partner Survey 2

Questions	WC Response	SN Response	PG Response
I park a distance from my destination to walk more.	Rarely	Rarely	Sometimes
I take the stairs instead of the elevator.	Rarely	Sometimes	Often
I look forward to the weekend so I can move about outdoors in fresh air and sunshine.	Often	Rarely/Sometimes	Sometimes
I do some form of exercise daily.	Always	Sometimes	Always
When I exercise, I feel less depressed.	Sometimes	Always	Never
I am willing to learn more about how I can make exercise a part of my life.	Yes	Yes	Yes

ercise, and movement. A tool based on the traditional genogram, utilized by many family counselors, was developed for this purpose. The traditional genogram was expanded by the author to obtain family background on sport, exercise, and movement. Each participant completed the Sport/Exercise/Movement Genogram with a rating according to the participant's perception of the significant person (or pet) activity level. Participants rated the person over the lifetime.

DISCUSSION OF WC SPORT/EXERCISE/ MOVEMENT GENOGRAM

The genogram was the basis for a discussion of the following:

1. The degree of activity of individual members in sport/exercise/movement followed by a description of the type of activities that generated the rating;
2. Cause and effect: Did parents influence children? Did siblings influence each other? Did patterns emerge? In what ways?
3. Did any members overeat, have anorexia, bulimia, or other?
4. Is there anything that you would like to change as a result of this exercise?

WC's mother was an "elite athlete," on the high school gymnastics team, and WC's "role model." Her mother maintained a high level of fitness with exemplary posture and a lean and muscular body into her eighties. WC stated that her father was "highly active" in high school playing some school sports. Later in life he became ill and sedentary. WC's sister was rated as "highly active." WC stated that she, herself, was "highly active" in her teens and young adult years, and attributed this to running with her dogs. Both parents influenced WC and her sister's activity level. They enjoyed outdoor activities as children. WC's sister overeats, and though active, is overweight. WC has a history of anorexia. Presently at 5'4," she weighs 120 pounds. Although WC presents as slender, she would like to lose additional weight. She walks her dogs daily. She has been encouraged to eat a more healthy diet.

DISCUSSION OF SN'S SPORT/MOVEMENT/ EXERCISE GENOGRAM

SN rated both parents moderately active since they enjoyed social dancing. She rated herself highly active prior to the onset of her schizophrenia, sedentary thereafter. Her sister was rated an elite athlete as a dancer. Her brother was moderately active. SN believed that her eldest son would be more active except for the fact that he spent so much of his time at the computer. Her younger son was rated moderately active. SN's parents influenced her sister and herself with regard to a love of dance. SN would have enjoyed going farther in the dance field, but circumstances in her life, marriage and her illness, made that dream impossible. SN has remarried a man who fractured his hip and is out of work. Once he recovers, she would like to do more activities with him.

DISCUSSION OF PG'S SPORT/MOVEMENT/ EXERCISE GENOGRAM

Initially, PG elected to "pass" on a discussion of her genogram. It was noted that she had a much easier time rating the family than herself. Later in the group session, she volunteered that she is constantly active "on the run" at work. She is exhausted when she returns and naps. Notably, she rated her two youngest children as approaching "elite athlete" status.

It was impossible not to be struck by the detail of information about feeling states within the family of origin which emerged from this exercise and the likelihood that a great deal of the information would not have been forthcoming absent the specific sport/exercise questioning.

GAMES AND GENERAL MOVEMENT

Games and play were a natural prelude to an introduction of movement, and provided an opportunity to observe and assess the groups' readiness for greater physiological demands. They were not only used as tools to measure and expand upon social interactions, but also as an opportunity for problem solving. Since games can be designed to be "safe," they met the most basic requirement for growth.

Dr. Marianne Torbert (1997), Director of the Leonard Gordon Institute for Human Development Through Play of Temple University, has observed:

> Movement activities are action based and observable. Not only the planner but also the participant is receiving immediate and constant evaluation feedback. Just as one learns muscular control

through frequent and repetitive experiences, such play can also be a tool to evaluate social interactions and to experience and deal with various emotional responses and personal feelings. (p. vi)

It was theorized that the "inner child" of each member required an arena where she could safely take chances and explore unused potential. Several action-oriented games were introduced throughout the sixteen week period. These included: (a) Categories, (b) an adaptation of "Mirroring" (Torbert, 1997), and (c) Bop-It. Generally, the games were played at the beginning of group as ice-breakers, stress and tension relievers, and team and rapport builders.

In the game "Categories," the leader selected a category (e.g., "Flowers" or "Flavors of Ice-cream"). A smiley face pillow was tossed in a circle from one member to another. When the pillow was caught, an example of one type within a category (e.g., rose or vanilla), was given. The game ended when all examples within a category had been exhausted. All members had fun with the game of Categories. There was laughing at the choices others made and general group support to keep the smiley pillow in motion. Everyone was able to catch the pillow and to think of numerous examples within a given category. This game accomplished the goals of releasing tension and anxiety, providing an opportunity for movement, and inclusion of all group members (Torbert, 1997). It relaxed the participants, and socially reinforced them as a group.

In an adaptation of "Mirroring" (Torbert, 1997), a leader presented a movement that was imitated by the others. Players rotated leading throughout the game with some interesting results. Since many of these women had some nervous movement, it was not immediately clear what movement was to be imitated. At times, it was hard to distinguish between deliberate movement and idiosyncratic motion. However, when mistakes were made, the women laughed or offered support. An example of the group support occurred when PG hesitated in moving as she did in speaking. She was offered the opportunity to pass, but persevered until she lead a marching movement. PG was clearly pleased with herself, and the group cheered her on.

"Bop-It" used a commercial toy by that name. It required coordination, auditory discrimination, and rhythm. The game is designed to be played individually, or in a group. There are three movements utilized in Bop-It; twisting, pulling, and tapping. On command, e.g., "twist-it," "pull-it," or "bop-it," a player had a measured time period in which to complete the motion. Play continued until failure occurred. A score of the number of successful completions was then given. Players tried to better their personal best in an individual version, or to keep the Bop-It in play by passing it on signal in a group version.

The game of Bop-It was not originally a planned activity. SN noticed the toy and began to experiment. Since PG was late for this session, SN and WC were encouraged to play. Due to the short response time, WC failed consistently. When PG entered group and observed WC's difficulty, she would not attempt the game. Clearly, Bop-It did not encourage inclusion, and was abandoned rather quickly.

INDIVIDUAL WALK-TALK THERAPY SESSIONS

As mentioned previously, since safety was the primary concern, walk-talk sessions were initiated with the utmost caution. SN was the first participant to engage in a walk-talk session. She was advised that the walk was geared toward her comfort level; she could return to the office at any time. Although sneakers were recommended, SN arrived for her first session in shoes with a slight lift. Since she did not think this would be a problem, we proceeded with a short walk. We passed no one along the way, and returned in about ten minutes time. There was no focus on timing or pace, just an easy walk with an opportunity to move and enjoy the fresh air.

The session prior, I had discussed daily exercise with SN. I suggested that she do just one set of knee lifts in the morning. As SN laughed, I told her, "a little bit of something is better than a lot of nothing." SN smiled as she revealed that she had done her knee lifts several times during the week, "when I remembered them."

SN did arrive with sneakers for her second session; we headed out immediately retracing our original route. She presented as much more hopeful about her future. During this session, she referred to a "visualization" about playing tennis with a friend. Her mood was positive with more vigor than usual. Following the walk, a change in mood was noted in my office as we processed her unhappy first marriage and the onset of her illness. Perhaps SN had reserved this weighty subject for the "shelter" of the office.

SN participated in two walk-talk sessions. She stated, "Something in me has changed in the past few weeks." One week after her first walk-talk session, SN reported walking a distance to meet her husband. Under ordinary circumstances "I would have just waited there for him to pick me up."

WC had one walk-talk session at the time of this writing. The twenty-five minute walk was easy given that she walks her dogs daily. WC inquired whether she could bring her smallest dog on future walks. Each of her pets have attended individual therapy sessions with her at various times, so including the dog was easily accommodated.

The benefits of walking were expounded to both WC and SN including the concept of greater "clarity of thinking and a capacity to synthesize in new ways" (Hays, 1999). Both the 25-minute walk with WC and the short ten minute walk with SN were difficult to assess, however, in this regard. Focus on these characteristics is planned for future sessions.

CLASS, RACE, ETHNICITY, AND SEXUAL ORIENTATION AS BARRIERS TO OR FACILITATORS OF TREATMENT

The genesis of the group of women with severe and chronic mental illness began with a need; the women were already clients of the referring psychiatrist and sport psychologist who recognized a need for group work as an adjunct to their psychiatric treatment and counseling service. At least two of the women's symptomatology bordered between out-patient treatment and needing more intensive intervention such as day treatment or inpatient services.

Thus, with this small case study of three heterosexual Caucasian women, there was no opportunity to examine class, race, ethnicity or sexual orientation as possible factors in the treatment. Without any measures for these factors, no claim can be made with regard to them as barriers to or facilitators of treatment. Class, race, ethnicity and sexual orientation, however, are desirable as components of a study assessing techniques to facilitate sport, exercise, and movement in the mentally ill. Hopefully, future research will include a more representative population of the mentally ill.

Participants in this support group were all of a lower socio-economic class; however, two of the three participants received some financial support from their families who were of a higher socio-economic class. This support helped them to access private psychiatric care and private counseling services. Given that the mentally ill are often dependent on community mental health programs, and that such programs focus on meeting minimal basic needs (McFarland, 1994), the women in this group had access to services not ordinarily available to a like population. Accordingly, the socioeconomic class of the families of two of the participants served as a facilitator in that they provided a greater access to treatment. Future studies in this area with a more diverse population are needed.

CONCLUSIONS

The primary goal of the women's group was to promote healing. The scope of this paper does not permit a discussion of the other modalities utilized nor the ways in which they may have enhanced, or detracted from, the use of movement and exercise techniques discussed in this paper.

Overall, two of the women made progress, no small feat in dealing with this client population. SN and WC committed to individual walk-talk sessions. Some changes with regard to movement and exercise were noted, e.g., SN reported visualizing herself playing tennis, and WC indicated she will stop smoking. Because of the liability of her psychiatric problems, PG could not consistently take advantage of an exercise regimen.

A major discovery was the importance of the judicious use of games. The Bop-It game was not successful from the viewpoint of inclusion and in building self-esteem. Clearly it was beyond the level of coordination possessed by WC. PG flatly refused to play the game. Noting the reactions of the others, SN's initial enthusiasm was dampened.

A challenge throughout was the wide difference in attitude, background, and interest in movement. Although PG was the youngest participant, with a self-rating of "moderately active" on the sport/exercise/movement genogram, the symptomology of her avoidant personality disorder often precluded even "easing into" an activity. It was not unusual for her to present in a "catatonic-like" state, almost frozen in a blank stare and wringing her hands. It was initially easier to engage her in art therapy, games, and crafts, her first loves, than in movement. She stated that exercise "never" relieved her depression.

By the time of the second interview, the group had become more accustomed to movement and games. After "Categories" SN noted perspiration and laughed about how tossing a pillow had been the cause. Given her decline from "highly active" (when she engaged in swing dance, skiing, skating and volleyball) to her current "sedentary" life style, the message SN received with the pillow toss was that she desperately needed to recondition herself.

All of the group members responded positively to the games of "Categories" and "Mirroring." These games provided opportunities to move in a variety of ways. As leaders, some of the members did small side bends or twists. Others stretched and alternated various muscle groups.

Breathing patterns changed; they discharged tension. All of the participants were energized by these two games.

Attitudes toward the various techniques varied among the participants. PG displayed little interest in any of the sport/movement/exercise activities with the exception of some games, and persisted that exercise "never" relieved depression. She contrasted markedly from the other two women who displayed greater interest in the partner interviews, the genogram, and consented readily to walk-talk sessions. However, the group remained supportive regardless of an individuals' interest or desire to participate in selected activities. Accordingly, screening by interest and/or ability may be neither practical nor desirable in some settings.

It was observed that games were received with varying attitudes ranging from a desire to play and have fun to wanting to sit them out. Given that games can be constructed to provide a sense of safety and inclusion as well as an appropriate level of challenge, the basic needs of the group participants should be factored into their selection.

Given the initial inertia of some of the participants, the group activities, e.g., partner interviews and sport/movement/exercise genogram, leading up to movement and walk-talk sessions appeared to be effective. Two women remarked on the insights gained from these discussions, and were motivated to begin walk-talk sessions. Although the duration of these sessions was inadequate for any substantive physiological change, their initiation broke through SN's state of inertia, and triggered visions of a more active time in the lives of both SN and CW.

The number of sessions actually fully devoted to sport/movement/exercise was not adequate to explore this new modality with depth. Work with such disordered clients always poses great difficulty in sequencing and continuity. The sessions experienced, however, had numerous positive outcomes. All three women indicated that they would be interested in receiving educational information regarding the benefits of exercise and mental health. I have hopes that the observations made during this group can serve as an underpinning for further work in this area and with these women.

REFERENCES

Andreasen, N. C. (1994). Introduction. In Backlar, P., *The family face of schizophrenia*. (pp. 27-41). New York: A Jeremy P. Tarcher/Putnam Book, G. P. Putnam's Sons.

Brewer, B. W. & Petrie, T. A. (1996). Psychopathology in sport and exercise. In Van Raalte, J. L. & B. W. Brewer (Eds.), *Exploring sport and exercise psychology*. (pp. 257-274) Washington, DC: American Psychological Association.

Brown, R. S. (1987). Exercise as an adjunct to the treatment of mental disorders. In Morgan, W. P. & S. E. Goldston (Eds.), *Exercise and mental health*. (pp. 131-137). New York: Hemisphere.

Buffone, G. W. (1997). Running and depression. In M. L. Sachs & G. W. Buffone (Eds.), *Running as therapy: An integrated approach*. (pp. 6-22). Northvale, New Jersey: Jason Aronson.

Greist, J. H. (1987). Exercise intervention with depressed outpatients. In W.P. Morgan & S.E. Goldston, *Exercise and mental health*. (pp. 117-121). New York: Hemisphere.

Harris, D. V. (1987). Comparative effectiveness of running therapy and psychotherapy. In W. P. Morgan & S. E. Goldston, *Exercise and mental health*. (pp. 123-130). New York: Hemisphere.

Hays, K. F. (1999). *Working it out: Using exercise in psychotherapy*. Washington, DC: American Psychological Association.

Kostrubala, T. (1997). Running and therapy. In M. L. Sachs & G. W. Buffone (Eds.), *Running as therapy: An integrated approach*. (pp. 112-124). Northvale, New Jersey: Jason Aronson.

Martinsen, E. W. (1987). Exercise and medication in the psychiatric patient. In W. P. Morgan & S. E. Goldston, *Exercise and mental health*. (pp. 85-95). New York: Hemisphere.

McFarland, B. H. (1994). Commentary on a father's story: Learning to live with schizophrenia. In Backlar, P., *The family face of schizophrenia*. (pp. 56-82). New York: A Jeremy P. Tarcher/Putnam Book, G. P. Putnam's Sons.

Millman, D. (1992). *No Ordinary Moments: A peaceful warrior's guide to daily life*. Tiburon, California: H. J. Kramer.

Rejeski, W. J., & Thompson, A. (1993). Historical and conceptual roots of exercise psychology. In P. Seraganian (Ed.), *Exercise psychology: The influence of physical exercise on psychological processes* (pp. 3-35). New York: Wiley.

Sachs, M. L. & Pargman, D. (1997). Running addiction. In M. L. Sachs & G. W. Buffone (Eds.), *Running as therapy: An integrated approach*. (pp. 231-252). Northvale, New Jersey: Jason Aronson.

Sime, W. E. (1987). Exercise in the prevention and treatment of depression. In W. P. Morgan & S. E. Goldston, *Exercise and mental health*. (pp. 145-152). New York: Hemisphere.

Sime, W. E. (1996). Guidelines for clinical applications of exercise therapy for mental health. In J. L. Van Raalte & B. W. Brewer (Eds.), *Exploring sport and exercise psychology*. (pp. 159-187). Washington, DC: American Psychological Association.

Summers, J. & Wolstat, H. (1997). Creative running. In M. L. Sachs & G. W. Buffone (Eds.), *Running as therapy: An integrated approach*. (pp. 93-100) Northvale, NJ: Jason Aronson.

Torbert, M. (1997). *Follow me*. Philadelphia: Leonard Gordon Institute for Human Development Through Play of Temple University, Philadelphia.

Narrative Therapy:
Inviting the Use of Sport as Metaphor

Jackquelyn Mascher

SUMMARY. The benefits of exercise and sport extend far beyond the physical and emotional to the socio-psychological, metaphysical, global, and historical. One way to introduce and maintain sport as a therapeutic tool is to do so metaphorically, using narrative-sport therapy. That is, in addition to the introduction of physical interventions, a narrative approach to therapy is well suited to stretch exercise to its fullest meanings. Exercise and sport are powerful possibilities for women in therapy. A woman's story of herself as sporting can also be a powerful language for transformative (therapeutic) experience. In this article, some of the major tenets of narrative therapy are explained using stories from women's lacrosse specifically, and for women who exercise in general. This article uses the concepts of history-making, boundaries, reflecting, and networking to illustrate only a few of the many possible productive intersections of sport and narrative therapy. *[Article copies available for a fee from The Haworth Document Delivery Service: 1-800-HAWORTH. E-mail address: <getinfo@ haworthpressinc.com> Website: <http://www.HaworthPress.com> © 2002 by The Haworth Press, Inc. All rights reserved.]*

KEYWORDS. Narrative therapy, women, exercise

Jackquelyn Mascher is affiliated with Boston College.

Address correspondence to: Jackquelyn Mascher, Institute for the Study and Promotion of Race and Culture at Boston College, Campion Hall, 140 Commonwealth Avenue, Chestnut Hill, MA 02467 (E-mail: mascher@bc.edu).

The author wishes to thank Jodie Kliman, PhD, for her personal and professional resources.

[Haworth co-indexing entry note]: "Narrative Therapy: Inviting the Use of Sport as Metaphor." Mascher, Jackquelyn. Co-published simultaneously in *Women & Therapy* (The Haworth Press, Inc.) Vol. 25, No. 2, 2002, pp. 57-74; and: *Exercise and Sport in Feminist Therapy: Constructing Modalities and Assessing Outcomes* (ed: Ruth L. Hall, and Carole A. Oglesby) The Haworth Press, Inc., 2002, pp. 57-74. Single or multiple copies of this article are available for a fee from The Haworth Document Delivery Service [1-800-HAWORTH, 9:00 a.m. - 5:00 p.m. (EST). E-mail address: getinfo@haworthpressinc.com].

INTRODUCTION

Exercise and sport are therapeutic modalities, the benefits of which extend far beyond the physical to the socio-psychological, metaphysical, global, and historical. One way to introduce and maintain sport as a therapeutic tool is to do so metaphorically. That is, in addition to the introduction of physical interventions, a narrative approach to therapy is well suited to stretch exercise to its fullest meanings. Narrative therapy is a postmodern-feminist-constructivist approach that entails the co-construction of real, imagined, or possible stories of the past, present, or future. Narrative approaches are as much about the practice of therapy as they are about the histories and possibilities of therapy. Exercise and sport are powerful possibilities for women in therapy; women's stories of themselves as sporting can also be a powerful language for transformative (therapeutic) experience. By making exercise themes explicit as metaphor, a therapeutic relationship facilitates the bridging, not only a mind-body duality, but intrapsychic, interpersonal, and cross-cultural rifts as well.

Space considerations do not permit me to orient the reader more fully to the layered complexities of narrative therapy. Narrative approaches necessarily emerge from stories that are the participant's own. Partly because of this axiom of narrative therapy, and partly because of limitations inherent in writer-reader discourse, I illustrate narrative therapy approaches with some of my own stories. Thus, the purpose of this article is to orient readers to narrative therapy and to the possibilities of integrating sport and exercise with narrative therapy. Major assumptions of narrative therapy are presented along with ways in which sport-inclusive therapy may use such experiences as clinical metaphor.

NARRATIVE THERAPY: AN ORIENTATION

Narrative therapy is the name given to an approach that has been largely documented by White and Epston (1990). Narratives, or stories, are the principle metaphor in a therapy, and the therapeutic process is one of meaning-making. The stories themselves are re-produced and produced through discourse both in and outside of therapy. The themes of our stories are explanations for us. In narrative therapy, a 'problem' is often seen as a 'problematic story' which has power over a client. Problematic stories may become dominant (social, familial, cultural, historical, global) stories in the client's life. In part, narrative therapy becomes about the ways in which the client and the client's contexts (including the client's therapist) might come to externalize and then interact with, rather than internalize, these problematic stories. In therapeutic discourse occurring in or outside of a therapy session, narratives are remembered, re-remembered, mis-remembered, re-authored, and co-authored as part of the change process.

Narrative therapy assumes that: (a) realities are socially constructed, (b) realities are constituted through language, (c) realities are organized and maintained through narrative, and (d) there are no essential truths (Freedman & Combs, 1996). In essence, a person's lived experience is privileged in therapy while the therapist encourages multiple perspectives and deconstructs her own 'expert knowledge.' The therapist carries an assumption that change is always possible, and that there exist multiple and alternative stories in the face of dominating and problematic stories. The therapeutic process demands therapist self-reflexivity and accountability for his or her part in restraining any alternative stories that might continue to be hidden in therapy (Madigan & Law, 1998).

Narrative therapy is not merely a description, mirroring, or reflection of life events; nor is narrative therapy reductionist and fundamentalist in its meaning-making (White, 1995). Rather, the story metaphor is meant to be generative. Narrative therapy is not only about the deconstruction and construction of stories; it is about the interaction of stories that are at once representative, ironic, paradoxical, hierarchical, and deeply embedded in one another. Therefore, the practice of narrative therapy will depend on therapist narrative, client narrative, and the discourse that comes to be combinations of these narratives (Madigan & Law, 1998).

Narrative therapy calls attention to all dimensions of identity including class, race, ethnicity, and sexuality/orientation; dimensions that not only suffer from being traditionally marginalized in therapy but are routinely sidelined in sport contexts as well. It is no secret that exercise and sport continue to be realms of sexist, ableist, and racist contests, and that Western psychology is a practiced tradition that has perfected a masculinizing, objectifying, pathologizing, and skirting of critical social issues. However, rather than various dimensions of identity serving as barriers in therapy, narrative approaches personally, interpersonally, and sociopolitically empower clients. Narrative therapy can redefine psychological practice by giving fuller meaning to a woman's ability to exercise herself and by giving voice to her multiple identities.

True to a feminist narrative approach, I situate my discussion in the context of one of my own exercise activities, the sport of women's lacrosse. In this tradition, I firmly recognize my own compartmentalized psycho-socio-geographical history as a devoted athlete, quite separate from my other long-term salient identities as an upwardly mobile, White, lesbian, trauma survivor who studies issues of race and culture in counseling psychology. I want to integrate these identities with some of my most humbling, empowering, and lost identities as a former player on the United States women's lacrosse squad and former college coach. It is a healing exercise for me to explore ways in which I might bridge some of these competing identities and contested stories, and I am seeking to bridge my past (pre) occupations with my future career in counseling psychology. The ideas that follow may serve as templates for readers practicing a sport inclusive narrative therapy approach. However, my purpose in writing this article is not merely to present personal issues but for the ideas that follow to be mostly generative in the perceptions of the reader. In helping an athlete-client understand a dominant and problematic story, a narrative therapist leaves space for alternate and more helpful stories. With diverse clients, there may be an alternative exercise narrative that is helpful, or the discovery of an exercise narrative may be the alternative way of considering her experiences. The intensity or strength of sport in a client's life is not so important. Instead, sport inclusive narrative therapy is about how a client thinks of herself as a physical being and how she might exercise her self in private and political games. In a narrative approach to exercise and sport, contesting dichotomies are blurred. The stories that constrain us are categorical, and sport inclusive narrative therapy is about re-training ourselves and our body politic to transcend polarities (White, 1995) such as athlete/non-athlete or healthy/sick.

I will suggest some constructs and applications of a sport inclusive narrative therapy using one of my activities, women's lacrosse, as an example. I also provide examples of the sorts of questions a narrative therapist might use in order to address a problem and to facilitate change. The following sections illustrate the therapeutic concepts of histories, boundaries, reflecting, and networking. Using a narrative conceptualization, I address possible problematic stories in women's lacrosse specifically, and for women who exercise in general. However, these are only a few of the many possible productive intersections of sport and narrative therapy.

CO-CREATING HISTORIES

In a narrative approach, it is important to recognize that there are as many histories as there are selves, families, communities, and nations. Every client carries with her generations of stories that are her sources of strength, limitation, and adaptation. These storied and multiple selves, both experienced and possible, can be de-constructed and re-constructed (co-constructed) in a therapeutic setting. The continuities and changes that exist across these multiple identities are the foundations of a client's future experience. Getting a client to highlight preferred events and processes, or preferred details, can help her to make connections that together comprise a new and more helpful account of her past and future experience. Also, a therapist can help a client to identify which contextual elements of a story are connected with story outcomes to better understand change, and to form a "history of the present" for any particular client (White & Epston, 1990). This process can be broken down into three parts: defining a problematic story, externalizing a problematic story, and helping the alternative stories to emerge.

Defining the Problematic Story

Athletes, particularly females, may feel that it is inappropriate to speak of athletic experiences unless given permission, may feel such experiences are irrelevant, or may feel that exercise experiences are not powerful, expert, or accomplished enough to mention. Additionally, therapists may not have an ear for stories of exercise for many of these same reasons. However, because narrative therapists take a stance of not-knowing, inquiry about a client's very specific athletic experiences need not imply nor require that a therapist has expert knowledge in sport. A stance of not-knowing naturally fosters curiosity (Freedman & Combs, 1996).

In defining the problem, therapists must honor the client's experience and language that she uses to describe the problem. Even if the problem is thought to be a common one, the detailed experiences of the problems are unique (White, 1989) and definitions of the same problem in therapy are fluid and evolving. The problem can be defined specifically, in order to ascertain detailed effects of the problem, or the problem can be defined generally, in order to expand the perceived effects of the problem (White, 1989).

In narrative therapy, it is important to privilege the client's language of the problem. *Naming the plot* (Freedman & Combs, 1996) is empowering, as are all naming exercises, and may be particularly empowering for women around their physicality. A woman's ability to name herself, her injuries, and her experiences may be therapeutic in and of itself. Also, there may not be very much useful language for athletes to convey their sport experiences, and therapists simply cannot be familiar with all sports and exercises. As such, the following are questions that may be useful in defining a problematic story.

How many ways has your play been described? Do you find yourself questioning any of these descriptions? Are there ways in which coaches, trainers, or teammates have helped you feel worse about yourself? Do you think there is more to your athleticism than these descriptions? This thing you are telling me about, what can we call it? What keeps you from achieving these goals you've been telling me about?

Externalizing the Problematic Story

Externalizing a client's story creates the context in which a problem and a client can be perceived as separate entities, and so indicates that the client is not the problem (Madigan & Law, 1998). Externalizing also places a problem in the contexts of others so that it can be more clear how the problem affects people other than the client, and enables people to recognize and work together to overcome a problem. It is the externalizing discourse of narrative therapy that challenges individualistic views of problems and successes, allows for multiple versions of the same problem to exist, and avoids pathologizing clients. Rather than objectifying a client, externalizing language objectifies the problem at hand. For example, the following questions might be helpful in externalizing an athlete's debilitating anger:

Do others see your anger? What are the effects of the anger in your life? What does this 'anger' look like during play? How is it that the anger makes you lose your concentration? How are you different when the anger is with you? When does the anger get the best of you? When did you first come to notice anger?

One way to structure these externalizing conversations is through relative influence questioning (White, 1989). With these questions, clients are asked to describe the influence that the problematic story has on their lives, but clients are also asked to describe the influence they have on the life of the problematic story. Therapists can also inquire how the problem affects the client's relationship with herself and with others. Part of externalizing the problem is defining the dynamic, bidirectional relationship the client has, and others have, with the problem:

What effect does this anger have on your life? Does the anger affect others? How does the anger know to approach you? Would you expect a teammate to treat you this way? Does anyone or anything in your life help the anger along? Does the anger have a game plan? What is your relationship to anger? Has anger helped you in the past? Are there ways that you invite the anger in, or ways that you dismiss it?

Part of externalizing and contextualizing stories about a woman's physical activity is, of course, acknowledging that there are contextual institutionalized restraints on her lived experiences. Just as feminist therapists validate normal development in the context of maladaptive social institutions and narcissystems, narrative therapists can acknowledge storied struggles within these same systems. In the sport of lacrosse, there are two, relatively distinct, varieties: the "women's game" and the "men's game." As various pressures emerge today for one form for males and females, the women's game is often perceived to be endangered. A client, having deep "stories" as a female lacrosse player, may benefit from the explication of this storied history.

Most clients will not know the political histories of their sports. But narrative therapists can assume that subjugating histories exist, and can be transparent with regard to their positioning on these cultural issues (Madigan & Law, 1998). Therapists can assume that there are multiple layers of history, and can assume that women have stories of their physical selves. Individual and community based versions of personal history intersect with political and social histories, and so intersect with the development of an athletic program or sport.

Even if such a complex history remains hidden to the client and the therapist, and is not engaged in therapy, it is an absent yet implicit theme (White, 2000). The narrative therapy model of power assumes that sources of power are often invisible to those who experience it most intensely, that such power isolates the people it subjugates, and that it is difficult for people to discern when they being subjugated and when they are not (Epston & White, 1992). Still, a narrative therapist can assume that her client's story is situated in these multiply embedded layers whether or not they have been, or will be, discussed. The client's story is a map generated by these various versions of history, and so holds keys to her multiple layers of development.

Defining the Alternative Stories

Sport inclusive narrative therapy requires that therapists listen for versions of lost or silenced exercising histories. If descriptions of sport, exercise, or other physical experiences have not been initiated by a client in therapy, then it may be necessary to actively listen for these omissions. For example, silenced sport history might mean a new way for a woman to think about her physical self, a new way of interacting with officials or teammates, or realizing some of her lost stories of esteem and success. Exercise itself may be a personal exception to oppression, a story of strength, a reclaiming of a physical self, and an expression of self. Asking a client for an account in which she exercised might help her to unite some of her compartmentalized selves in a past struggle, externalize a problem with which she has been engaged, or create new languages for her struggles. In addition, alternative stories can place her struggles in the context of broader social discourses in a way that combats isolation, identifies her social groups, and invites intersections with the stories of others. The recognition of new exercise narratives can foster empowerment in a client that extends far beyond the satisfaction that comes from physical activity alone.

Clients can be helped to understand the ways in which others' stories have restricted them. Recognizing such dominant discourse is a valuable therapeutic exercise. Therapists can also assume that there is a relationship between the silenced stories and the silencing stories; therapists need to be actively listening for their own and their client's internalized discourses that suppress other, more liberating stories. On multiple levels, silenced stories are indicators of the dominating and oppressing stories that need to be elucidated via a series of deconstructing questions.

In deconstructing a dominating story, therapists need to work to define unique history outcomes, and unique accounts of these outcomes. Such unique outcomes can be found in the relationships between the client and the problem, or between others and the problem. To achieve this, therapists can help clients review the history of a problem, with a focus on experiences that contradict the client's normal experience of the dominant story in the past, currently, or in the future. In the case of a deeply self-deprecating athlete, possible alternative stories can emerge via the use of questions such as the following:

Can you recall a time when you could have submitted to the demands of self-hatred, but did not? Was there anything you did to prepare yourself for this? Did you recognize the significance of this achievement at that time? What was the difference between your experience then, and your experience now? Are you surprised by your ability to deal with your self-hatred differently right now? What could you do to check your self-hatred the next time it approaches? How did you come up with these ideas? How will you feel differently when you check your self-hatred?

Negative explanations (White, 1989) are themes that have been re-strained by a dominant explanation of a client's experience. In other words, our dominating life themes occur because these are unrestrained compared to alternative themes and experiences. These are the alternatives that, in the face of our problematic stories, may seem untenable or unrealistic.

What is it that would cause your self-hatred to occur, despite the fact that others don't feel this way about you? Can you remember qualities of yourself that your self-hatred made you forget? What keeps you going, despite the self-hatred? What rules do you break in order to get away from the self-hatred? Who would be amazed at your ability to escape it? When/Where/With whom are you most free from it? What is it about the way women's lacrosse players are supposed to be that keeps you from talking about this self-hatred? When you choose to remain silent, what does this say about your internal strength, and does that fit with an idea of weakness or strength?

In most cases, the unique outcomes and the negative (silenced) explanations are themes of resilience and adaptiveness, which, when strung together, create a new story line about the client. New techniques, or metaphors for these techniques, can be the basis for life skills yet to be developed; in addition, an athlete-client's old techniques can be exercised in new ways. The coping skills that clients have are the ones that may not get talked about, but that need to be recognized as a client's ability to be adaptive in stressful situations. These life, or athletic, skills can come from watching others, or they can be a mark of a client's uniqueness and creativity. For athletes, the narrative metaphor can come from their sports experiences. For example, there is a specific technique in women's lacrosse called cradling that is a necessary movement in order for a player to run and maintain possession of the ball at the same time. This movement tends to be idiosyncratic to each player, and is developed by imitating another, by experimenting in different situations, and by practicing what is comfortable. Therapeutically, this particular technique can take on a new, even nurturing, meaning for a client:

What motivates you to move differently? Does your ability to nurture come naturally, or did it take practice? Does your ability to take care of things under pressure surprise you/others? How, exactly, did the cradling help you escape/put you in a different position? Do you think that your response to the stressful situation was making it more or less likely for the problem to continue? Did it take imagination for you to cradle yourself out of trouble? Is there more than one way to cradle, especially if you feel threatened? Do you cradle when you don't feel threatened?

Instituting Boundaries

From the onset, a therapeutic relationship is a differently powered one. Power differences also exist in race, ethnicity, gender, sexuality, able bodiedness, and other dimensions. In addition, the realms of exercise and sport continue to be bastions of sexist, ableist, and racist contests, and these contests exist economically, administratively, and programmatically. These differences in power result in differential unearned privileges and access to resources, a particular problem for women and marginalized people in sport. It is a hallmark of narrative therapy that such boundaries are intended to be acknowledged, and that these dimensions of difference in or outside of a therapy session can be made explicit, whether they exist between therapist and client or the client and others.

Narrative therapists should be sensitive to such boundaries, and to the differences of power that determine what is valid in a field of discourse. Refereed contests, including therapy sessions, involve explicit and implicit rules and regulations such as time, place, function, language, and so on. Many narrative and feminist therapists would acknowledge boundaries as necessarily messy, variable, and shifting continually. In sport, as in therapy, the contested realities of relationships can involve the negotiating of a beginning/end, cost/benefit, offensive/defensive, and dependence/independence.

For example, in the women's lacrosse experience, the field of play is determined in part by the natural boundaries of the area. While the goals are placed at a specified distance from one another, and while there are some markings on the field, external boundaries are negotiated with each play. Rather than pretending that there are no legitimate boundaries, referees use their power and flexibility explicitly with the interests of players, onlookers, and historical circumstances in mind. The boundaries become obvious when the players or witnesses are in danger; using their own intuition, interpretation, and experience, those who are empowered to blow the whistle do so when a play becomes non-productive or harmful.

Although the above description of the nature and function of boundaries is highly specific to women's lacrosse, therapists can help clients find their own metaphors and language for boundary issues. The boundary metaphor describes her experience on the field, in life, and in therapy. In any case, the theme might be dominant and subjugating, or it might be alternative and helpful. These metaphors can be used as a language to help the therapist understand what bounds, by being made explicit, will be most helpful during therapy:

What are your expectations? What has been your past experience? Would you expect my role to be a monitoring or teaching one? What ideas about boundaries do you currently hold? Does anything in particular stand out to you as shaping these ideas? How might you explain your conflicting ideas about boundaries? How does what I've said affect our relationship/your view of me/of yourself? Have you ever acted outside of these limits? What did it take to do so? What possibilities does this open up for you and others?

Feminist and constructivist approaches recognize institutional constraints (Brown, 1994) and systemic barriers to forming diverse alliances. As therapists we need to acknowledge and validate these barriers to alliances, but we can also name our contributions to these barriers. Boundaries can be used (re)productively to decompartmentalize interpersonal and intrapersonal identities and integrate experiences. The contested boundaries between identities is a borderland that is often exaggerated, ignored or denied altogether. It is, however, an interactional space where the opportunity for change resides. This is the idea that "it takes at least two somethings to create a difference" (Bateson, 1980, p. 76).

In narrative therapy, such a change can come from a therapist raising dilemmas or contradictions (Epston & White, 1992; White, 1989) within or external to the problematic story. This requires recognizing boundaries, recognizing differences, then thinking in new ways. Thinking in new ways may require negotiating, cooperating, or inviting the observations of others. Therapists can also use dilemmas to assess a client's readiness for change. The following questions are dilemma-raising questions:

What message does this give you? Does it make you feel more or less safe? When do/don't you feel in control of this boundary? Do you feel controlled by the boundary, if so, when? How would bringing others in on this fear help you to see yourself as a whole person? What difference would this make in your relationship with yourself? Do you think that you should begin to defeat your fear, or should you continue to let the fear win? Do you think you should continue to let your fear score points on you? How has this new version of yourself as an athlete changed your future?

Reflecting

Reflecting refers to a narrative therapy technique, but it also refers rather specifically to movements and strategies associated with women's lacrosse. On the one hand, standard practice in narrative therapy includes the use of a 'reflecting team,' or participant-observers who process the therapeutic activity periodically during the course of a therapy session. On the other hand, reflecting in a sport is the process of matching another player in order to affect her strategies and decisions. More generally, reflection has two important elements: positioning and generating change. Explicit positioning often leads to authentic and interactive change.

Positioning

The phenomenon of explicitly locating or situating oneself is not new to feminist theorists in psychology, sociology, anthropology, and other fields. Narrative therapists take ethical positions, ones that afford marginalized clients a voice, ones that make the therapist's own positions clear with language, and they use language that indicates their position. Therapy is an invitation to interact so that a unique outcome can be generated, and therapists take positions that explicitly value the client's unique and preferred outcomes. In a narrative approach, speakers and relationships continually shift, and so it is important to name biases and interpretations in an ongoing way. Narrative therapists, from a position of not-knowing, can join with the client not so much innocently as transparently (Freedman & Combs, 1996; Madigan & Law, 1998; White, 1995).

Therapists can ask story development questions (Freedman & Combs, 1996), for example, about the process, details, time, context, and people of a story to help make a client's position clear. In addition, Freedman and Combs suggest asking meaning questions. That is, genuine inquiry about a client's meaning-making, characteristics and qualities of relationships, hopes, values, beliefs, and knowledges facilitates the process of a client situating herself (White, 2000):

What ideas in our culture support your dominance? Submission? I normally take a stand for non-self-injurious behavior. Can you see how I might arrive at this position? What do you think of my/your position? How does this position affect our work together? Do you have questions for me regarding my position? May I ask you questions regarding your position? (Are you/Am I) aware of the events from my own history that are informing my position?

Positioning is what Haraway (1998) calls situated knowledges. One's position in therapy, and/or on a playing field, grounds one for interaction. A client's perception of her own position is critical to her interactions with others on the field and on the periphery. Positionings are relationships that occur fluidly and continually. Even the labels of a practiced position (a name during a contest, e.g., wing, center, goalie) or role (what others expect of you, such as a gender role, e.g., mother) evolve. There are changes and continuities in positions within one play as well as across contexts and time, and with increased flexibility and sophistication, players can come to understand, relate to, and enact multiple positions. Unique redescription questions (White, 1989) ask clients to assign significance and consequences to these unique outcomes and accounts:

What does this tell you about yourself now? What do these developments tell me about you as a person? What is the most significant thing we've talked about today? What have you learned about yourself/our relationship/the problem? What do you think I see, as your therapist? What do you think I've noticed to lead me to feel this way?

Generating Real Change: Mirroring as an Illusion

A narrative approach to reflecting assumes that there are multiple ways to perceive events, or that it is anti-therapeutic to merely parrot another's 'mother tongue' (Brown, 1994). Reflection (even self-reflection) has the potential to maintain hierarchical and oppressive structures under the guise of change. Mirroring is an empty reflecting, and it is a deceptive patriarchal tool born of psychoanalysis and not-so-distant medical traditions. Non-therapeutic mirroring occurs when a therapist fails to situate herself. Therapists who take a stance of knowing, neither inquiring nor encouraging clients to inquire about positioning, pathologize and label a client's experience. The therapist who assumes to know–or assumes that he should know–the nature of an exercise experience is not a narrative therapist. The narcissism of the omniscient therapist produces nothing short of a sports complex–an intricate pathological arena that only increases the distance between a therapist and a client, or a client from her interactive spectators.

A narrative stance, however, assumes that there is no perfect positioning or mirroring because narratives are dynamic and interactive. Therefore, a therapist's reflections about herself, her clients, and her processes with her clients can never be truthful and factual. Reflecting about others includes reflecting about oneself but, additionally, it involves situating all of this reflecting in one's own experiences:

Which parts of the clients' story gain my attention? How do I understand the fact that my attention is drawn to some narratives instead of others? In what ways might I inadvertently contribute to the client's problematic story? In what ways can I maintain awareness of the power our society has given me?

However, such therapist self-reflections, should they become increasingly routine and private, risk becoming mirrored affirmations, just as reflecting a client's concerns back to her does little to change the reality of her problematic situation. There is a distinction between passive reflecting (of self or others) and active reflecting, or interacting for change. Reflexivity is not enough "for escaping the false choice between realism and relativism . . . what we need is to make a difference" (Haraway, 1998, p. 16).

For example, a mirroring skill in lacrosse can be a hapless defensive tactic. Interactive mirroring, however, can dictate, is reactionary, is anticipatory, and consequential. In a field sport, at times, when another team has control of a game, advocating for oneself requires a change in the nature of the game. A more active approach is sometimes required to change the outcome of an experience. In any case, for therapy or exercise, a shift of positioning can dramatically affect the outcome of an event.

The active mirroring in narrative therapy is akin to Haraway's (1998) idea of how change occurs. Rather than reflexivity, Haraway adopts the idea of diffraction, or the bending of information. In other words, the therapeutic psychologist cannot merely and passively reflect back to the client, and also cannot merely self-reflect. Real changes, or shifts, occur in an interaction that minimizes gaps between participants:

How do you think this has changed my picture of you as an athlete or person? What will your teammates/coach discover about you that they may have not seen? What does this tell others about you? Can you see how much this means to me, that you have taken this step? What does this mean for your relationship with your exercise? What is it like for you to see this new version of yourself? If you were to accept this new vision of yourself, what would be your next step?

Working the Net in a Non-Traditional Way

Relationships in narrative therapy, like other feminist and constructivist approaches, are central to goals. In the interactional spaces of relationships there is collaboration and a co-creation of multiple goals and processes. In narrative therapy the storytelling, itself, is a political action. Shared storytelling can extend beyond the therapy room to the creation of networks that are critical to the development of a client, of systems, and of movements. In the listening and observing of stories about physical selves, exercise becomes a productive relational canvas in therapy. "Working the net" is used here as an athletic metaphor for a goal, the area around a goal, or movement toward a goal. More obviously, "working the net" refers to the use of collaborative networks to achieve a desired outcome. Networking is a non-traditional approach to therapy in many ways (elsewhere called 'network therapy'), but networking for female exercisers may be especially critical to generate support and shared experience through relationships and witnessing.

Emphasizing Relationships

Narrative therapy focuses on client relationships, both with people and with problematic and helpful stories. Of course, these relationships undergo countless revisions, and can have multiple meanings. The therapist might invite a history of friendships in or around teams and organizations. In addition to interpersonal relationships, clients might provide narratives about their relationships with exercise itself, for example, or talk about how other relationships were affected by participation in exercise activity. A history of relationships might highlight family tensions, or personal and collective activism of team members engaged in a radically female sport that resists masculinization. Although collaboration, sharing, and respect are not uniquely female, the recognition of these elements of teamwork is a profoundly feminist act. Sport metaphors in therapy can engender flexibility, the strength and endurance of pain tolerance, and a collective autonomy of finesse and intelligence that is traditionally female.

Sometimes, numerous relationships converge around central topics for clients, and this can be profoundly helpful. For example, the relationships of myself with the sport of women's lacrosse, women's lacrosse with its Native American origins, my exercised political self with my sporting physical self, my silence with my voice, myself with my girlfriend, and other relationships for me all carry a theme of oppressed sexuality. In other words, there is an obvious silencing of lesbian identities, particularly in women's sports by popular media; to an extent, these subjugating systems in the United States are the same ones that colonized Native lacrosse traditions. There is a flexibility of same-sex affiliation and the absence of any distinctly gendered roles on female athletic teams that is reminiscent of Native 'two-spirited' or berdache peoples. I do not mean to confuse Native societies with postmodern sexual rhetoric, but there is something familiar about European misunderstandings of Native sexualities on the one hand, and widespread contemporary heterosexist discourses on the other hand.

A hallmark of narrative and feminist approaches is the inclusion of interpersonal relationship-based collaboration. Collaboration can occur at all levels and for all involved. Ethically, of course, therapists might consider having consultants and supervisors at the ready, but it is also critical to help a client network for the purpose of establishing more direct support systems and witnesses. When a client's support systems are fortified, by extension, so are a therapist's. White (1995) has written of one particular therapeutic technique of forwarding correspondences from one client to another with the purpose of facilitating a therapeutic exchange and shared knowledges.

With the introduction and maintenance of sport as a therapeutic tool, narrative therapists might expand the ways they think about realms of networking, in a sense, like political bodybuilding. Consultations might be conducted with people in administrative positions, former teammates, rivals, or coaches. Athletic activities, in addition to the institutions affiliated with athletic activities, have their own unique and complex political histories. Of course, these politics are inextricably related to broader social, political, and historical contexts; therapists' network relationships can be as multiply layered and complex.

Acts of Witnessing

As with all stories, there is power in an act of witnessing. Witnesses do not provide clarity and objectivity in an exercise; rather, witnesses are participatory. Narrative therapists might make use of what Haraway (1998) calls the 'modest witness,' an honest public subjectivity that mobilizes and motivates change. Stories are continually reconstructed in the collection and recollection of those bearing witness, so that stories become shared experiences as they are perceived, dismembered, remembered, and mis-remembered before, during, and after an event. The witnessing itself becomes a gaze-worthy spectacle, so that the direction of shared experiences runs in multiple directions. Witnesses draw from and contribute energy to an event, thereby joining with each other, and possibly motivating the exerciser. All of those on a sideline, spectators, athletes, and others participate and can gain a sense of self from watching a collaborating team or an exercising woman.

Whether narrative therapists use individual or team approaches, and whether exercise is solitary or communal, audiences can be acknowledged. Clients might consider it helpful to recruit their audiences from time to time. By asking about a client's network, the therapist can assess support for the client, or accumulate a collaborative strength and is more likely to see silenced themes or stories: What stories would others share with you if they were here?

Within the context of a particular sport or exercise a narrative approach emphasizes the relationship of variables to one another, for example, de-emphasizing a 'starter' and a 'scorer' as primary, but identifying and validating the contributions of the more invisible members of a team. As another way of forging relationships with intrapersonal or interpersonal subjugated identities, the client can come to appreciate the whole of herself or her exercising experience (including those who are around her). In addition, the client's acceptance of herself as a witness to others may also decenter her problems and make it easier to invite real or imagined others to collaborate.

CONCLUSIONS AND RECOMMENDATIONS

This article has focused on sport as a powerful metaphor, and on the multiply layered possibilities of using exercise concepts in combination with narrative concepts. Narrative approaches can facilitate the introduction and maintenance of exercise in a practiced and literal sense as well, but the introduction of sport as metaphor allows more general discourse about imagined, real, possible, discovered, and productive identities. Some story possibilities in sport inclusive narrative therapy might be the pursuit of alternative versions of history, the meaning of boundaries, active reflecting, and expansive networking.

Narrative concepts work best in combination with other approaches, and should be considered in light of continued changes to feminist theory and dynamic feminist philosophies. With any technique and theory, therapists risk perpetuating dominant discourses or illusory change, but more widespread use of basic narrative techniques will help feminists shift from categorical treatments to relational interventions. In this article, I have allowed possibilities for a narrative sport therapy model to emerge from a broad feminist therapy theory (Brown, 1994) and cyberfeminist theory (Haraway, 1998). Such combinations in therapy, however, will be co-constructed and re-constructed idiosyncratically.

REFERENCES

Bateson, G. (1980). *Mind and nature: A necessary unity.* New York: Bantam.

Brown, L.S. (1994). *Subversive dialogues: Theory in feminist therapy.* New York: Basic.

Epston, D., & White, M. (1992). *Experience, contradiction, narrative & imagination.* Adelaide: Dulwich Centre.

Freedman, J., & Combs, G. (1996). *Narrative therapy: The social construction of preferred realities.* New York: W.W. Norton.

Haraway, D.J. (1991). *Simians, cyborgs, and women: The reinvention of nature.* New York: Routledge.

Haraway, D.J. (1998). Modest_Witness@Second_Millennium.FemaleMan(c)_ Meets_ OncoMouse(tm): Feminism and technoscience. New York: Routledge.

Madigan, S. & Law, I. (Eds.). (1998*). Praxis: Situating discourse, feminism & politics in narrative therapies.* Vancouver: The Cardigan Press.

Maguire, J. (1999). *Global sport: Identities, societies, civilizations.* Malden, MA: Polity Press.

White, M. (1989). *Selected papers.* Adelaide: Dulwich Centre.

White, M. (1995). *Re-authoring lives: Interviews and essays.* Adelaide, Australia: Dulwich.

White, M. (2000). *Reflections on narrative practice: Essays and interviews.* Adelaide: Dulwich Centre.

White, M. & Epston, D. (1990). *Narrative means to therapeutic ends.* New York: Norton.

APPLICATIONS FROM SPORT PSYCHOLOGY AND EXERCISE SCIENCE

Promoting Exercise Compliance: A Cognitive-Behavioral Approach

Karen L. Hill

SUMMARY. Exercise is a stressor. It raises both heart rate and blood pressure. It re-routes blood flow toward working muscles and away from functions such as digestion and reproduction. It pours energizing, sympathetic nervous system hormones into the blood stream and pushes the physiology of the body above normal limits into uncomfortable and sometimes even painful states. This challenge to the body, and the accompanying discomfort, acts as a catalyst for emotional and psychological, as well as physical, stress.

The Cannon-Bard theory posits that responses to stress are the well-known "fight-or-flight" (Cannon, 1932) responses. Under the stress of

Karen L. Hill is affiliated with Pennsylvania State University, Delaware County.

Address correspondence to: Karen Hill, PhD, Associate Professor, The Pennsylvania State University, Delaware County Campus College of Health and Human Development, Department of Kinesiology, 25 Yearsely Mills Road, Media, PA 19063 (E-mail: klh7@psu.edu).

[Haworth co-indexing entry note]: "Promoting Exercise Compliance: A Cognitive-Behavioral Approach." Hill, Karen L. Co-published simultaneously in *Women & Therapy* (The Haworth Press, Inc.) Vol. 25, No. 2, 2002, pp. 75-90; and: *Exercise and Sport in Feminist Therapy: Constructing Modalities and Assessing Outcomes* (ed: Ruth L. Hall, and Carole A. Oglesby) The Haworth Press, Inc., 2002, pp. 75-90. Single or multiple copies of this article are available for a fee from The Haworth Document Delivery Service [1-800-HAWORTH, 9:00 a.m. - 5:00 p.m. (EST). E-mail address: getinfo@haworthpressinc.com].

exercise, individuals either flee–try to avoid–the stressor, which partially accounts for the low rate of long term compliance to exercise programs, or they get aggressive and determined–they "fight," primarily with themselves, to persist in the exercise or sport activity.

In *Biobehavioral Responses to Stress in Females: Tend-and-Befriend, Not Fight-or-Flight,* Taylor, Klein, Lewis, Gruenewald, Gurung and Updegraff (2000) recently identified an alternative interpretation of the body's stress response. This stress response is described as the "tend-and-befriend" model, and early indicators show it may be a preferred pattern of stress response by females. This paper describes the tend and befriend model and suggests how it might be applied therapeutically to exercise and sport activities for women. *[Article copies available for a fee from The Haworth Document Delivery Service: 1-800-HAWORTH. E-mail address: <getinfo@haworthpressinc.com> Website: <http://www.HaworthPress. com> © 2002 by The Haworth Press, Inc. All rights reserved.]*

KEYWORDS. Stress, exercise compliance, women

EXERCISE AS A STRESSOR

"My heart started to pound, I was gasping for breath and sweating profusely. My knees felt weak and my stomach was queasy." How would you perceive a client reporting these experiences? Fearful? Panic-stricken?–Certainly under some form of stress. It is interesting to note that these symptoms are common physiological responses to exercise, although psychologists seldom view exercise as a stressor. In fact, exercise is often viewed as a stress-reliever rather than a stressor. Paradoxically, both perspectives of exercise are valid. In order to understand how exercise is a stressor and a stress-reliever, it is necessary to examine the most basic exercise physiology findings in regard to the acute and chronic effects of exercise on the body (Wade & Baker, 1995).

When an individual begins a single bout of exercise, one of the first adjustments made by the body is vasodilatation–an opening up–of the blood vessels that channel blood-borne oxygen and nutrients to the muscle tissues that are starting to work. This systemic increase in the volume of the blood vessels serving the muscles would, by itself, cause blood pressure to drop quickly leading to dizziness or unconsciousness; however, other changes in the body prevent this from happening. These other changes are vasoconstriction–or closing–of blood vessels serving the digestive and reproductive systems, as well as an increase in cardiac output as the heart contracts more frequently. With the increase in cardiac output, respiratory effort increases to oxygenate the blood, and the individual begins to breathe more frequently and more forcefully. The metabolic energy that fuels the exercise session accelerates the body's demand for glycogen and results in changes in blood sugar levels. The increased metabolic activity also generates heat and the body begins to sweat as a cooling mechanism to dissipate the heat. These responses are mediated by the autonomic nervous system as the sympathetic complex prepares the body for increased work capacity by stimulating the adrenal medulla to secrete catecholamines into the bloodstream. Consequently, the acute physiological responses to exercise actually mimic physiological indicators of other types of stress-pounding heart, breathlessness, sweating, and butterflies in the stomach due to slowed digestion. These physical experiences are viewed as uncomfortable, and sometimes even as alarming, by many people. Individuals who exercise regularly are not alarmed by these physiological signals during exercise because they have habituated to them. However, individuals who have little experience with exercise may experience various degrees of alarm with the onset of these body signals and experience emotional stress– from fear or anxiety of the unknown–as well as the normal physical stresses of the exercise experience.

Unlike circumstances with other forms of stress that may be unavoidable, the physiological stressors associated with exercise cease when exercise is halted. The body gradually returns to homeostasis and the individual is released from the stressor. This sense of release, or negative reinforcement, can serve to condition some people to exercise and contributes to exercise compliance. However, if individuals associate the negative reinforcement with stopping exercise, it can condition them to avoid exercise.

If individuals persist in exercise, they habituate to the acute stressors of the exercise activity and are rewarded by the chronic responses to exercise. Long-term physiological responses to exercise include increased work capacity, decreases in resting heart rate and blood pressure, and other adaptations that make the cardiovascular and respiratory systems more efficient. Additionally, there is often an increase in muscle mass, decrease in body fat, decrease in muscular tension, and increase in strength and endurance that accompanies long-term compliance to an exercise program. These physiological changes are beneficial to overall health and the prevention of heart disease, obesity, hypertension, diabetes and osteoporosis, as well as other chronic ailments. The long-term physical adaptations to exercise increase the capacities of the body and actually enable the body to withstand higher levels of stress. In other words, habitual exercise increases the body's capacity to handle the physiological aspects of stress. Through the training effect, exercise uses acute stress to gradually increase the capacity of the body to handle higher levels of stress. Exercise is a short-term stressor that results in chronic stress relief because it increases the capacity of the body to handle stress. The stress reducing properties of a well-designed exercise program primarily result from the training that accompanies long-term compliance to a progressively more intensive exercise load. The body adapts to handle the increased loads and becomes more resistant to stressors (Dishman, 1982).

Unfortunately, in order to reap the chronic beneficial effects of exercise, one must get past the acute stress responses that accompany exercise activity, and most Americans fail to do this. Three out of four Americans do not exercise regularly (Puretz, Haas, & Meltzer, 1997), and 50% of Americans who initiate an exercise program quit within 6 months (Dishman, 1982). In the fight-or-flight stress response model, it appears that the "flight" option is the choice of the majority of Americans. One in four Americans have found ways to "fight" the acute stresses of exercise and do so on a regular basis, but three of four flee from extended exercise programs. The American Heart Association "Statement for Health Professionals by the Committee on Exercise and Cardiac Rehabilitation of the Council on Clinical Cardiology" maintained the following: "it is important to develop strategies to improve exercise initiation and adherence, especially for persons who are among the least active–some African-American women, the less educated, the obese, and the elderly" (Fletcher, Balady, Blair, Blumenthal, Caspersen, Chaitman, Epstein, Sivarajan Froelicher, Froelicher, Pina, & Pollock, 1996, p. 2). Women constitute a disproportionate percentage of these inactive groups.

Interventions to improve exercise compliance must take into consideration the fight-or-flight response to stress induced by single bouts of exercise. There is another model of stress response, however, and perhaps by designing exercise programs with this model in mind, in addition to providing interventions to deal with fight-or-flight tendencies, we can increase the chances of some individuals, and women in particular, to successfully deal with the acute stresses of exercise so they can enjoy the chronic benefits.

TEND-AND-BEFRIEND STRESS RESPONSE

While extensive research has been done on fight-or-flight stress responses, most of the fight-or-flight studies have used male subjects. Prior to 1995, women comprised only 17% of participants in laboratory studies of physiological responses to stress. Furthermore an examination of 200, post-1985, studies of physiological and neuroendocrine responses to an acute experimental stressor shows only 34% of the participants were female (Taylor et al., 2000). Justification for the exclusion of females in stress studies has been that women's monthly cyclical variation in neuroendocrine responses has produced inconsistent results regarding fight-or-flight responses in females. Taylor et al. recently proposed that perhaps the equivocal nature of the female data on fight-or-flight patterns "is not due solely to neuroendocrine variations, but also to the fact that the female stress response is not exclusively, nor even predominantly, fight-or-flight" (p. 412).

Taylor et al. (2000) suggest that while women may physiologically respond to stressors with a fight-or-flight response, behaviorally, females responses to stress are characterized more by tend-and-befriend patterns. "Tending involves nurturant activities, designed to protect the self and offspring, that promote safety and reduce distress; befriending is the creation and maintenance of social networks that may aid in this process" (Taylor et al., 2000, p. 411). Tending behaviors involve a wide variety of activities including calming behaviors such as kissing, soothing, touching, caressing, verbal calming statements, caretaking behaviors such as feeding and grooming, and shielding behaviors such as hugging. Befriending behaviors include affiliation behaviors such as inviting, showing acceptance, conversing and attending to another in a supportive manner.

The tend and befriend model is based on (a) evolutionary, (b) neuroendocrine, and (c) affiliation patterns associated with women. The evolutionary rationale for the tend-and-befriend theory is based on the assumption of female prominence in caretaking. Because women are initially heavily invested in infant survival through pregnancy and lactation, natural selection should favor not only survival of the woman herself, but also of her children. Fighting or fleeing are viable strategies for survival but these actions have disadvantages for women with children. Fighting puts the woman in danger and her death or incapacitation makes survival of her young children unlikely. Fleeing is difficult with young children and would be a slow and often unsuccessful strategy. These disadvantages suggest that alternative strategies for dealing with the stress of threat may have developed especially for women (Taylor et al., 2000). Behaviors that maximize the likelihood of survival of both mother and child in threatening situations are tending behaviors such as quieting and caring for children that allow them to blend into the environment and hide. Likewise befriending behaviors that increase ones resources by banding together (strength in numbers) would also be a workable strategy for survival of self and offspring. The evolutionary argument for tend-and-befriend responses suggests that tend-and-befriend behaviors would become hard-wired into females through natural selection favoring conservation of what works best.

Neuroendocrine support for tend-and-befriend stress response is also related to caregiving activities. Taylor et al. (2000) "propose that the neurobiological underpinning of the attachment-caregiving system provide a foundation for this stress regulatory system. Specifically, oxytocin and endogenous opioid mechanisms may be at the core of the tend-and-befriend response" (p. 412). Oxytocin is a hormone released from the posterior pituitary gland that plays a role in childbirth and lactation by causing smooth muscle to contract in the uterus and release of milk during lactation. Animal studies have shown that oxytocin also has a role in pair bonding, mate-guarding and social memory (Medicine Net.com, 2000). Oxytocin is associated with parasympathetic responses that tend to relax and restore the body to homeostasis. Both males and females release it in response to stress, but females tend to have greater response rates. Oxytocin release during stress is suppressed by androgens and its effects are enhanced by estrogen, suggesting why it appears to impact stress responses more for women than men (Taylor et al., 2000).

The literature in sociology and social psychology also supports the behavioral tendency for women to affiliate in response to stress. Social learning and cultural roles support women's caregiving and affiliation behaviors and "the 'befriending' pattern is one of the most robust sex differences reported in the literature on adult human behavior under stress" (Belle, 1987; Luchow, Reifman, & McIntosh, 1998 as cited in Taylor et al., 2000). Additionally, in studies of sex differences regarding motivation in sport and exercise programs, females have identified affiliation as a more significant factor than males for participation in exercise (Gill, Williams, Dowd, & Beaudoin, 1996) and the importance of affiliation during exercise appears to increase for women as they age (Gill & Overdorf, 1994). While Taylor et al. acknowledge limitations regarding the female propensity to favor tend-and-befriend responses to stress over fight-or-flight response, there is ample evidence supporting tend-and-befriend responses to stress in females to consider this response when promoting exercise programs to women.

EXERCISE AND STRESS MANAGEMENT

There are two major strategies for dealing with stress. One strategy is to attempt to reduce or eliminate the source of the stress. This is often referred to as stress reduction. In the case of exercise, stress reduction is counterproductive because it implies the cessation of exercise itself as exercise causes a stress response. A second strategy is stress management, which involves using coping mechanisms to attenuate the stress.

The exercise/sport experience can be organized to accommodate both "fight-or-flight" and "tend-and-befriend" stress responses through stress management. It is necessary to consider both patterns of response because individuals vary in their responses to stress and the nature of exercise is both physiological and behavioral. The physiological stresses of exercise have been outlined earlier in this paper. They are concerned primarily with the acute aspects of exercise. The behavioral aspect of exercise centers on the fact that exercise must be done consistently over time with programmatic specifications–it needs to be a chronic behavior and is a lifestyle change. Consideration of stress management techniques that address both patterns of stress response optimizes the chances for successful compliance to the exercise regimen.

PRE-EXERCISE CONSIDERATIONS

Before suggesting that a client begin an exercise program, several important issues must be addressed. The first issue is the current health of the client. The client must be examined for any organic contraindications to exercise. A thorough physical examination and consultation with a physician should proceed initiation of any exercise program by a sedentary individual. In addition to testing for cardiovascular and circulatory diseases, a complete physical clearance to exercise will identify and accommodate conditions, such as asthma and diabetes, which are directly affected by exercise. Furthermore, support from the client's physician in the form of encouragement to exercise may bolster motivation and remove any thoughts of threat to the health of the client due to exercise.

A second issue that should be examined prior to suggesting exercise to a client is the client's experience with exercise and her attitudes toward physical activity. Exploring questions such as "Has she exercised before?," "What physical activities does she enjoy?," "What activities did she enjoy as a child?" and "Does she view exercise positively or does it have negative implications such as being unfeminine?" Prior experiences and attitudes toward physical activity are the starting point for preparing to exercise. If a woman's views of exercise are negative, cognitive reframing should precede the initiation of an exercise program. Some common misperceptions associated with exercise are that it is unfeminine, inappropriate for older people and painful. These attitudes should be modified prior to starting a program or addressed within the first phases of a program to avoid interference with compliance of the program. Women who have little experience with exercise are also likely to experience more stress when initiating an exercise regimen. This new experience may make them feel out of control, they may be unable to properly interpret bodily sensations associated with exercise, and they may have doubts about whether their personal resources can match this new challenge. It is important to address these concerns and explain to the client what she might expect to experience during an exercise session.

While personal histories play a role in shaping the amount of stress perceived by individual women entering a physical activity program, another issue of concern is the client's individual stress stereotype. Stress stereotype refers to an individual's unique response to stress. While we all respond with the same general physiological markers–increased heart rate, blood pressure, muscular tension, vasodilation/vasoconstriction and temperature variation–the degree to which each one of these factors dominates the stress response varies from person to person. Some individuals are predominately vascular responders (blushing, nausea), some are muscular tension responders (tension headaches) and others may be cardiorespiratory (pounding heart, breathlessness) or temperature (sweating) responders. The extent to which exercise mimics a person's stereotypical stress response will temper the degree of alarm reaction experienced by the novice exerciser. For example, a woman who typically responds to stress with muscular tension may not be alarmed by a beginning aerobics dance class where muscular tension is kept low by the rhythmic, flexible and flowing movements of the dance. Another woman who is primarily a cardiorespiratory responder, however, may have to deal with the alarm of increased heart rate and some breathlessness early in the workout. The cardiorespiratory responder may be more successful if she begins her exercise program with a strength-training program that does not provoke the high degree of cardiorespiratory stress associated with aerobic programs. After several months of adjustment to strength training, aerobic training may be added in small, incremental steps to her exercise regimen. This training protocol offers the woman an opportunity to begin exercise with minimal engagement of her stress stereotype sensations, which might reduce the alarm experienced from the new exercise program. Of course it is impossible to avoid all of the physiological responses associated with stress when exercising because, as stated before, acute exercise is a stressor. However, some attention to the matching of the design of a new exercise program to counter the stress stereotype of the exerciser might serve to reduce the alarm experienced by the individual and make the initiation of activity less threatening.

Another issue of concern prior to initiating an exercise program is the timing of introducing this new stressor into the client's life events. Unless the client has previously habituated to an exercise activity or clearly views exercise as eustress, due to previous experience with sport and exercise, it is best to introduce an exercise program when other stressors and changes in the client's environment are low or decreasing. The reason for considering the client's current stress level is that stress is summative, and adding a new stressor to the client's life while other stresses are high may be counterproductive. The Holmes and Rahe (1967) Social Readjustment Rating Scale (formerly called the Life Events Scale), which is used to measure cumulative stresses of life changes, rates "Revision of personal habits" as the 29th largest stressor and assigns 24 points out of a possible 100 (for Death of a Spouse) to this life event. The view that stress is cumulative has been supported by research, and high scores on the Life Events Scale have been consistently associated with subsequent illness (Smith, 1993). Consequently, adding the burden of exercise stress onto a client who may be highly stressed from other life events is not always advisable.

A direct relationship between cumulative stress and exercise behavior was shown in a study in which 82 community-residing women kept exercise and stress diaries for eight consecutive weeks. In this study "during weeks with a high frequency of stressful events, participants exercised for less time and reported lower self-efficacy for meeting upcoming exercise goals" (Stetson, Rahn, Dubbert, Wilner & Mercury, 1997, p. 515). The women also exercised on significantly fewer days, omitted more planned exercise sessions, were less satisfied with their exercise and had lower self efficacy for meeting exercise goals during weeks of high perceived stress (Stetson et al., 1997). It appears that adding the acute stress of a new exercise program to the agenda of a person who is already under great stress is counterproductive. Additionally, it sets up a situation in which compliance to the new exercise program is less likely, especially for novice exercisers.

If the client is an individual who has experienced the stress-reducing properties of exercise due to previous participation in sport and exercise, giving up exercise will be stressful. Individuals, who view sport and exercise participation as "good stress" or stress-relieving, should be encouraged to continue to exercise. On the Social Readjustment Rating Scale, abandonment of an established exercise routine constitutes a "revision of personal habits." With individuals who have exercised regularly, an abandonment of exercise will increase stress. Not only will they miss the physical relief from exercise to which they have been accustomed, but they are likely to be cognitively stressed and emotionally upset because they are not getting their routine exercise participation.

EXERCISE AND TENDING

Taylor et al. (2000) presents evidence that suggests that women who are under stress often cope behaviorally by becoming more nurturing and caring toward their children. Studies by Repetti (1989, 1997) indicate that fathers who had highly stressful workdays (that did not include interpersonal stress) tended to withdraw from their families; however, mothers showed more nurturance and care on days of highest stress at work. Children reported that acts of affection–hugging, kissing, touching–and caregiving from their mothers were highest on the days that the mothers reported high stress at work. One possible explanation for this behavior is that caring physical contact (e.g., hugging, touching) promotes the release of oxytocin which invokes parasympathetic responses to combat the physiological strains of stress (Taylor et al., 2000). The sport/exercise research literature also supports the positive role of tending in contributing to exercise compliance. For example, including children or caring for a dog as part of an exercise program was designated as "enablers" of walking programs for older African American and American Indian women (Henderson & Ainsworth, 2000). This may be true for other female populations as well. If some women manage stress by tending to their children, then perhaps exercise programs should be shaped to accommodate this coping behavior.

One way to include tending into exercise programs for women with children is to design programs that women can do with their children. Women can engage in a walking program with small children by using strollers, and it is possible to engage in running programs with new strollers designed specifically for jogging. Cycling in a safe area with a child seat offers another opportunity to engage in physical activity with a child. "Mom and Tot" exercise or swimming programs, often available at local health clubs and Y's, provide another alternative for engaging in fitness with children. Older children can be involved with mom's exercise program too. A brisk walk, playing a round of golf or tennis with the children is fun and provides an opportunity for mother and child to talk and bond. Additionally, given the poor physical condition of many American children, 9 to 15% of whom are overweight, exercising with children promotes an active lifestyle for the child, too.

If a woman who is prone to respond to stress with tending behaviors cannot work out with her own children, seeking volunteer opportunities in programs like First Tee (a PGA program that introduces inner city children to golf) provides an opportunity to be philanthropic as well as exercise–a double "feel good" experience. Running or walking with the family dog is also an opportunity to exercise and care for another creature. With creativity and awareness of the needs and situation of the client, an exercise program that is designed to fit the lifestyle of a woman and provide tending experiences might have a better chance of becoming routine and allow the beneficial chronic effects of exercise to occur.

Recognizing the situation of the individual client prior to designing tending experiences in the exercise program is crucial, however. While some women will respond to stress with tending behaviors, many women who have small children would prefer to exercise without them because the exercise session gives them personal time and time to engage other adults. If trustworthy childcare is available and a woman prefers her exercise time to be personal time, it will be more rewarding for her to exercise without her children. However, for the many women who find that trustworthy, affordable childcare is not consistently available (a stressor itself), including children is a viable alternative. Organizing the exercise experience to include children and reframing a woman's childcare concerns from a barrier to an opportunity to do good for both themselves and their children can increase the chances of successful inclusion of physical activity in a woman's lifestyle.

EXERCISE AND BEFRIENDING

Taylor et al. (2000) state that one of the most robust gender differences in adult human behavior is the desire of females to affiliate during times of stress. Luckow et al. (1998) analyzed gender differences in coping by examining 26 affiliation/stress studies and found that only one study showed no differences between men and women on desire to affiliate under stress, but 25 studies favored women's desire to affiliate under stress. Given the strong evidence for women's preference to affiliate under stress, befriending response to exercise stress should be incorporated in physical activity programs by including affiliation opportunities in the design of exercise.

The opportunity to affiliate during stressful conditions may partially explain why aerobic exercise classes in dance, step, spinning, and even non-traditional activities like kick-boxing, are attractive to women. While men participate in these group classes, women participants usually substantially outnumber men participants. These organized classes have the advantage of setting aside a specific time in one's daily schedule for exercise in addition to providing opportunities to affiliate with other women. Health clubs and YMCAs almost always include these group activities in their offerings for women and joining this type of class enhances compliance. Research by Schachter (1959) suggests that women's affiliation preferences under stress are to associate with other women. Women who are new to exercise are likely, therefore, to feel more comfortable when joining a class that is comprised primarily of women. Compliance can be further promoted if the women in the exercise group know each other. Therefore, taking an exercise class with a friend, neighbor or co-worker enhances the appeal of the activity. Church sponsored aerobic classes in which the women know each other and have common ties could also enhance chances of long-term maintenance of activity programs. Exercising with a female friend who has similar physical capacities is important if both women are to benefit physically and be able to bond. It is difficult, for example, for joggers who exercise at different speeds to converse and connect. Therefore, the individual physical capacities of the women must match if affiliation is to be part of the exercise experience. It is also beneficial if the women share a liking for a particular exercise activity. Playing golf, tennis, softball or basketball with other women who also share enjoyment of these sports increases each participant's enjoyment by socially reinforcing each woman's choice of sport.

While women tend to prefer to associate with other women under stress, there are some women who may choose to exercise with an athletic male friend or partner. Some difficulties may arise with mismatches in size and skill level regardless of gender. Longer legs, differences in size and strength can interfere with necessary conditions for affiliation. For example, even when speed walking or jogging, outside formal competition, the pace may be so demanding that the client gets winded and is unable to converse. This eliminates a vital function for connection and a primary means of fulfilling affiliation objectives. Other problems may occur with unstructured co-ed or single-sex team sports such as soccer, basketball and softball. If the majority of the group has advanced skills in these sports, the client may have trouble getting beyond feeling inferior and out of place. This adds psychological stress to the exercise program. Additionally, some women may have increased fears of injury in a sport when many males or larger athletic women participate and, again, psychological stress is added to an already physiological stressful situation. There are some women who are challenged and benefit from participation with more skillful and experienced players in their sport. For a woman who is just beginning an exercise regimen, however, exercising with like-skilled people, especially other women, has both physiological and social advantages.

Hays (1999) suggests that psychologists might walk or jog with their clients as part of therapy. This idea has great value, for it enables the therapist to reassure the client that their acute responses to exercise are normal, and it provides an opportunity for affiliation by associating exercise with the intimacy and open sharing experienced during therapy. The exercise/talk session allows the client to immediately address any issues surrounding the exercise experience that may be bothersome or disconcerting. It gives the psychologist opportunities to not only allay fears but also to project in both word and by example that exercise is a positive, rewarding activity.

ORGANIZING WOMEN'S PHYSICAL ACTIVITY TO ACCOMMODATE FIGHT-OR-FLIGHT PATTERN

This paper views exercise from the perspective of stress theory, specifically from the tend-and-befriend stress theory (Taylor et al., 2000) recently proposed as a preferred response of females to stress. While there is evidence that many women preferentially respond to stress using tend-and-befriend behaviors which release the calming hormone oxytocin, and provide social support to deal with the stressful situation, fight-or-flight responses almost certainly accompany tend-and-be-friend responses to new exercise programs. Therefore fight-or-flight responses must also be considered in exercise stress. There are numerous cognitive-behavioral techniques to address the fight-or-flight response, as this response theory has been the centerpiece of stress theory for the past 70 years. Systematic desensitization, visualization, behavioral contracting, and goal setting are time-tested techniques for encouraging life-style changes. For example, addressing the fight response of dealing with exercise stress often entails changing an individual's approach to exercise from "something I dread but have to force myself to do anyway," to emphasize the play and enjoyment aspect of exercise. It entails re-thinking and planning exercise as joyful play rather than as a personal chore and as something to look forward to rather than something over which to anguish. Emphasizing the playful aspects of exercise, the freedom of movement, the enjoyment of nature can be accomplished by selecting an exercise mode that incorporates these qualities for the client. The mode of exercise, whether it is riding a bicycle like when you were a child, or walking in a park and noticing the beauties of nature, should invoke positive and even joyful feelings. Returning to some childhood activities, such as jumping rope, scooter riding and skating can be progressively incorporated into exercise programs to increase a sense of play and joy with movement. For individuals with diminished capacity, an activity such as swinging on a playground swing can be a playful introductory exercise activity. (If the client feels self-conscious, she can take a child along and swing together.) In addition to selecting a playful activity with the client, it is important to set up a progressive program, so that the client is not overly strained during a single bout of exercise. For beginning exercise activities, the physiological effort should not exceed the point where the client cannot carry on a conversation while performing the exercise. As physiological capacity increases, exercise intensity will also increase, but the rule-of-thumb that the client should be able to talk during the activity prevents over-exertion and will keep post-exercise muscle and joint soreness to a minimum. It also contributes to the ability to tend or befriend an exercise partner.

The flight response to exercise is a bit more problematic, and, as mentioned before, it is one of the major responses in that people tend to quit or give-up on exercise programs. One reason for the strength of the flight response is that quitting an onerous exercise is usually negatively reinforcing, and operant conditioning increases the tendency to stop exercising. One way to counteract this operant conditioning is through cognitive awareness. Cognitive awareness has been shown to interrupt operant conditioning. For example, in a treatment for alcoholism in which the alcoholic beverage is spiked with nausea-producing chemicals, the treatment often fails to curb alcohol consumption if the alcoholic is cognitively aware that the added chemical, and not the alcoholic drink, is the cause of the nausea. Similarity, using cognitive awareness to an advantage in activity compliance by alerting individuals about the inherent stress response as the body begins strenuous exercise can help combat its effect. Additionally, planning some positive reinforcement for exercise compliance, such as having a massage after exercising faithfully for a period of time or even receiving a tee shirt after completing a program, might promote persistence in the activity program.

CONCLUSION

This paper views acute exercise sessions as a physiological, and sometimes psychological stressor and posits that continuous exercise behavior is a major lifestyle change for sedentary women. It views women's responses to exercise in light of their reactions to other sources of stress especially tend-and-befriend reactions and fight-or-flight reactions. This paper is based on assumptions that have some basis in research evidence but have not been directly empirically tested under conditions of exercise stress. Future research is needed to ascertain whether exercise programs that are designed to include opportunities for tend-and-befriend behaviors enhance compliance preferentially for women.

Techniques to counteract fight or flight stress response patterns, such as behavioral contracting have received more research attention primarily due to the domination of this stress theory. None of the techniques that deal with fight-or-flight stress responses are mutually exclusive with tend and befriend considerations, and until further research is forthcoming, using techniques that allow for both responses to exercise stress may enhance compliance, especially for women.

REFERENCES

Belle, D. (1987). Gender differences in the social moderators of stress. In R. C. Barnett, L. Biener, & G. Garuch (Eds.) *Gender and Stress* (pp. 257-277). New York: The Free Press.
Cannon, W. (1932). *The wisdom of the body*. New York: Norton.

Dishman R. (1982). Compliance/adherence in health related exercise. *Health Psychology, 1*, 237-267.

Fletcher, G., Balady, G., Blair, S., Blumenthal, J., Caspersen, C., Chaitman, B., Epstein, S. Sivarajan Froelicher, E., Froelicher, V., Pina, I., & Pollock, M. (1996). *Statement on Exercise: Benefits and Recommendations for Physical Activity Programs for All Americans: A Statement for Health Professionals by the Committee on Exercise and Cardiac Rehabilitation of the Council on Clinical Cardiology,* American Heart Association. Retrieved Sept. 26, 2000 from the World Wide Web: http:///www.americanheart.org/Scientific/statements/1996/0815_exp.html

Gill, D., Williams, L., Dowd, D., & Beaudoin, C. (1996). Competitive orientations and motives of adult sport and exercise participants. *Journal of Sport Behavior, 19*, 307-318.

Gill, K., & Overdorf, V. (1994). Incentives for exercise in younger and older women. *Journal of Sport Behavior, 17*, 87-97.

Hays, K. (1999). *Working it out: Using exercise in psychotherapy.* Washington, DC: American Psychological Association.

Henderson, K., & Ainsworth, B. (2000). Enablers and constraints to walking for older African American and American Indian women: The cultural activity participation study. *Research Quarterly for Exercise and Sport, 71*, 313-321.

Holmes, T., & Rahe, R. (1967). The social readjustment rating scale. *Journal of Psychosomatic Research, 11*, 213-218.

Luckow, A., Reifman, A., & McIntosh, D. (1998, August). Gender differences in coping: A meta-analysis. Poster presented to the annual meetings of the American Psychological Association, San Francisco, CA.

MedicineNet.com., Medical References. Retrieved September 26, 2000 from the World Wide Web: http://www.medicinenet.com/Script/Main/Art.asp?li=MNI&ArticleKey=13789:

Puretz, S., Haas, A., & Meltzer, D. (1997). *The woman's guide to peak performance.* Berkeley, CA: Celestial Arts. p. 17.

Repetti, R. (1989). Effects of daily workload on subsequent behavior during marital interactions: The role of social withdrawal and spouse support. *Journal of Personality and Social Psychology, 57*, 651-659.

Repetti, R. (1997, April). The effects of daily job stress on parent behavior with preadolescents. Paper presented to the biennial meeting of the Society for Research in Child Development, Washington, DC.

Schachter, S. (1959). *The psychology of affiliation.* Stanford, CA: Stanford University Press.

Smith, J. (1993). *Creative stress management.* Englewood Cliffs, NJ: Prentice Hall.

Stetson, B., Rahn, J., Dubbert, P., Wilner, B., & Mercury, M. (1997). Prospective evaluation of the effects of stress on exercise adherence in community-residing women. *Health Psychology, 16*, 6: 515-520.

Taylor, S., Klein, L., Lewis, B., Gruenewald, T., Gurung, R., & Updegraff, J. (2000). Biobehavioral responses to stress in females: Tend-and-Befriend, Not Fight-or-Flight. *Psychological Review, 107*, 411-429.

Wade, M.G., & Baker, J.A. (1995*). Introduction to kinesiology: The science and practice of physical activity.* Madison, WI: Brown and Benchmark.

Effect of an Exercise Program
on Quality of Life
of Women with Fibromyalgia

Namita Gandhi
Karen P. DePauw
Dennis G. Dolny
Timothy Freson

SUMMARY. The purpose of this study was to examine the effect of a 10-week/20-session exercise program on quality of life (QOL) of women with fibromyalgia (FM). Thirty-two women with FM participated in one of the following groups: hospital-based group (G) (n = 10);

Namita Gandhi is affiliated with Integrative Movement Clinic and Albany General Hospital. Karen P. DePauw is affiliated with Washington State University. Dennis G. Dolny is affiliated with the University of Idaho. Timothy Freson is affiliated with Washington State University.

Address correspondence to: Namita Gandhi, 6310 NW Concord Drive, Corvallis, OR 97330 (E-mail: namitagandhi@yahoo.com).

Thanks to the Gritman Medical Center, Moscow, ID for providing the facility for conducting this research and to Jean Sweetapple, PTA for volunteering her time to do the measurements. Very special appreciation and thanks are extended to all the research participants for volunteering their time and precious energy.

A portion of this research was presented at the American College of Sports Medicine Northwest chapter annual conference in Boise, ID on March 17, 2000 and won an outstanding Student Research Award. This research was approved by the Washington State University Institutional Review Board for the protection of human subjects. Written informed consent was obtained from all the research participants.

[Haworth co-indexing entry note]: "Effect of an Exercise Program on Quality of Life of Women with Fibromyalgia." Gandhi, Namita et al. Co-published simultaneously in *Women & Therapy* (The Haworth Press, Inc.) Vol. 25, No. 2, 2002, pp. 91-103; and: *Exercise and Sport in Feminist Therapy: Constructing Modalities and Assessing Outcomes* (ed: Ruth L. Hall, and Carole A. Oglesby) The Haworth Press, Inc., 2002, pp. 91-103. Single or multiple copies of this article are available for a fee from The Haworth Document Delivery Service [1-800-HAWORTH, 9:00 a.m. - 5:00 p.m. (EST). E-mail address: getinfo@haworthpressinc.com].

home-based group (H) (n = 10); non-exercising control group (C) (n = 12). The hospital-based exercise program was conducted twice per week, and the home-based group participants followed the videotaped exercise program and maintained a detailed exercise log. The measures used assessed the participants' subjective and objective quality of life. Twenty-one women met all the completion requirements for the study. The baseline age (years) means were: C = 43.50 (n = 8), G = 51.78 (n = 9), H = 56 (n = 4). Data were analyzed using a one-way ANOVA. Over the ten-week period, significant improvements were made in the Range of Motion and in the Fibromyalgia Impact Questionnaire scores of the two exercise groups. However, the Tender Point Count and Tender Point Severity scores did not show any significant improvements. We conclude that the Fibromyalgia Exercise Program was effective in improving QOL of women with FM with minimal post exercise discomfort. *[Article copies available for a fee from The Haworth Document Delivery Service: 1-800-HAWORTH. E-mail address: <getinfo@haworthpressinc.com> Website: <http://www.HaworthPress.com> © 2002 by The Haworth Press, Inc. All rights reserved.]*

KEYWORDS. Chronic pain, pain management, range of motion, tender points, flexibility, breathing, relaxation, women

INTRODUCTION

Fibromyalgia (FM) is a condition predominately involving muscles and myofascia, and is *the most common cause of chronic, widespread musculoskeletal pain* (Bengtsson, Backman, Lindblom, & Skogh, 1994; Burckhardt, Clark, & Bennett, 1991; Goldberg, 1989; Henriksson, Gundmark, Benstsson, & Ek, 1992; Hiemeyer, Lutz, & Menninger, 1990; Starlanyl & Copeland, 1996; Wolfe, 1986). *According to the American College of Rheumatology (ACR), FM affects 3 to 6 million Americans. In 1987, the American Medical Association recognized FM as a true illness and a major cause of disability* (Starlanyl & Copeland, 1996).

Due to widespread muscular pain, persistent fatigue, multiple tender points, generalized stiffness and non-restorative sleep, individuals with FM find it extremely difficult to exercise (Bakker, Rutten, & Santen- Hoeufft, 1995; Bennett, 1994; Bennett, Burckhardt, & Clark, 1996; Burckhardt, Clark, & Padrick, 1989; Burckhardt, Mannerkorpi, Hedenberg, & Bjelle, 1994;

McCain, 1986; Mengshoel, Komnaes, & Forre, 1992; Natvig, Bruusgaard, & Eriksen, 1998). Most individuals with FM show signs of deconditioning due to prolonged inactivity (Bennett, 1994; Burckhardt, Clark & Bennett, 1993; Burckhardt et al., 1989). Studies have shown that as a result of impaired endurance, FM patients have a reduced quality of life (Burckhardt et al.,1991; Mengshoel et al., 1992; Natvig et al., 1998). The complex pathophysiology of fibromyalgia syndrome and the lower participation rate of FM patients in exercise programs have lead researchers to test several hypotheses (Van Denderen, Boersma, Zeinstra, Hollander, & Van Nerbos, 1992). Mengshoel (1990) reported that FM patients have normal aerobic capacity (aerobic capacity tested with a cycle ergometer test according to Aastrand's method and defined as O_2 ml/kg min) but reduced muscular strength. It has been demonstrated that there is no abnormality in the overall rate and pattern of utilization of oxygen during muscular exercise in FM patients (Sietsema, Cooper, Caro, Leibling, & Louie, 1993). A 20-week supervised cardiovascular training program for FM patients reported significant improvement in their cardiovascular fitness but no improvement in fatigue (McCain, Bell, Mai, & Halliday, 1988). Another study, with a very high dropout rate (~40%), showed improvement in dynamic endurance work for the upper extremities with no change in drug consumption in FM patients (Mengshoel et al., 1992).

Due to conflicting reports and a lack of exercise guidelines, it has been a challenge to design an effective exercise program for individuals with FM that will significantly improve their quality of life (QOL) without exacerbating their symptoms. Thus, the purpose of this research study was to design an exercise program that would enhance the QOL of women with FM.

METHOD

Participants

Thirty-two female FM patients ranging from 28 to 65 years in age participated in a 10-week study. Three groups were included in the study: a non-exercising control group (C) (n = 12), a hospital-based exercise group (G) (n = 10) and a home-based (videotaped exercise program) exercise group (H) (n = 10). Only women were included in the study because the Fibromyalgia Impact Questionnaire, a primary assessment tool, has only been validated using a female population (Burckhardt et al., 1991).

The participants in the study were solicited through three sources: the posting of flyers for the FM Exercise Program in local hospitals, doc- tors' offices and community centers; contacting an active FM Support Group in the area; and contacting participants of the FM Self-Help Course (sponsored by the Arthritis Foundation). The research design was quasi-experimental; hence, there was no random assignment of the participants. The FM Exercise Program flyer only contained the exer- cise program information and did not mention the home-based program or the control group. The home-based participants were solely solicited through the FM Support Group, and the controls were solicited through the FM Self-Help Course. There was no interaction among the three groups.

Before admission to the research project, the women were required to meet with the researcher at the Gritman Medical Center for an in-depth evaluation. The women's primary physicians were asked to complete and sign a Physician's Report confirming FM as the primary diagnosis and approving their participation in the FM exercise program. After the initial screening, 32 women with FM qualified and participated in the study. Written informed consent was obtained from all the participants in accordance with the guidelines set forth by the Washington State Univer- sity Institutional Review Board for the protection of human subjects.

Design and Procedure/Exercise Program

A 10-week/20-session exercise program was conducted from Octo- ber 1999 to December 1999. The hospital-based exercise program was conducted twice per week, every Tuesday and Thursday at the Gritman Medical Center. Each 1.5 hour long session consisted of 5 minutes of warm-up, 10 minutes of breathing and relaxation, 30 minutes of full body stretching, 10 minutes of strengthening, 15 to 30 minutes of aero- bic workout and 5 minutes of cool down. Home-based participants fol- lowed the program in a videotape format twice a week and maintained a detailed exercise log. The hospital-based participants exercised in a group setting, and the primary investigator personally lead all the exer- cise sessions.

Breathing and relaxation exercises included a guided systematic full body relaxation. Participants laid supine on a floor-mat and were en- couraged to use rolled-up towels and pillows to support the neck and lower back. The researcher guided the awareness of participants to body segments, systematically moving from head to toe. During these exercises, women were reminded several times to observe their breathing pattern and breathe diaphragmatically. In essence, women were taught to take a mental inventory of individual body segments and notice the painful parts before they started to exercise.

The stretching exercises were done mostly in sitting and lying positions in order to be better able to isolate the muscles that were being stretched while maintaining relaxation in other body segments. Included were a variety of traditional and non-traditional stretches. The recommended duration for holding the stretch was 0 to 30 seconds. The emphasis was on doing the stretches very slowly and with minimal discomfort. Women were asked to hold the stretch for as long as it felt comfortable and then very gently release it. If the participant had difficulty performing a certain stretch, the researcher modified the stretch. Women were given a five- to six-foot long flexible cord to help them with the stretching exercises. The cord was used mainly to stabilize the shoulder during the neck stretches and also to stretch the hamstrings in supine position. Again, women were constantly reminded throughout the session to breathe and relax.

The stretching was followed by the strengthening exercises, using Thera-Band (yellow). For every strengthening exercise, one set of ten repetitions was performed. Participants were advised to exclude the Thera-Band® exercises whenever pain levels were experienced as "too great."

For the aerobic workout, the hospital-based subjects used a combination of at least two to three different modes of exercise every time they exercised. The options were treadmill, bike with/without hand exerciser, stair-master and rowing (arms only, using the cord and a back of a chair). Participants were instructed to switch the mode of exercise to a different one (without any time-lapse) as soon as the involved muscle groups started to get fatigued. The most commonly performed combination was the bike with arms and the treadmill.

Materials/Assessment Instruments

Fibromyalgia Impact Questionnaire (FIQ). The FIQ was used in this study to measure the QOL improvement during the ten-week period (Burckhardt et al., 1991). The FIQ is a validated assessment and evaluation tool to measure the components of health status that are believed to be most affected by FM in the adult female population (Burckhardt et al., 1991). The FIQ is composed of 20 items. The first 11 items comprise a physical functioning scale. Each item is rated on a four point Likert-type scale. In items 12 and 13 individuals simply circle the number of days they felt well and the number of days they were unable to work because of FM symptoms in the past week. Items 14 through 20 are 10-centimeter visual analog scales marked in 1-centimeter increments on which the patient rates work difficulty, pain, fatigue, morning tiredness, stiffness, anxiety and depression.

Range of Motion. Bilateral range of motion (ROM) measurements of shoulder flexion, side-bend (spine flexion) and hip-flexion were done by a registered physical therapist assistant at the Gritman Medical Center. The goniometer was used to measure the degrees of flexion in the above mentioned joints/locations. Shoulder flexion and side-bend were done in a standing position and the hip-flexion was done in a lying down (supine) position with knees bent. Subjects were asked to stretch and warm-up the muscles before the measurements were taken.

Tender Point Count and Tender Point Severity. The American College of Rheumatology in 1990 Criteria for the classification of Fibromyalgia was used by the registered physical therapist assistant to perform the tender point examination (Wolfe, Smythe, & Yunus, 1990). A total of 18 tender points (bilateral/nine pairs) were evaluated by digital palpation, at a pressure of ~ 4kg. A 0 to 4-point scale was used to record the severity of tender points. Zero was no pain and four was unbearable pain. If the participant withdrew without palpation or refused to be touched at certain tender point locations, that was marked as four on the scale. A tender point had to be painful at palpation and not just "tender" to be rated above zero. All the tender points rated above zero were added for the tender point count (TPC) score. For the tender point severity (TPS) score the subject's individual scores for all the eighteen points were added together. The following bilateral tender point sites were examined: occiput, low cervical, trapezius, supraspinatus, second rib, lateral epicondyle, gluteal, greater trochanter and knee.

Index of Clinical Stress (ICS). The ICS was completed by the participants to measure the magnitude of problems with personal stress (Abell, 1991). The 25-item instrument is designed to reflect the range of perceptions associated with subjective stress. The ICS has documented internal consistency, with an alpha of 0.96.

Symptom Questionnaire (SQ). The SQ is a 92-item instrument with documented validity to measure four aspects of psychopathology and well-being (Kellner, 1987). It was completed by the women to evaluate depression, anxiety, somatization, anger-hostility, and also the four aspects of well-being: relaxed, contented, somatic well-being and friendly.

Quality of Life. In this research study, quality of life (QOL) was defined as a general sense of well-being based on participants' physiological and psychological parameters. Objective measurement included pretest and posttest scores on Fibromyalgia Impact Questionnaire (FIQ) completed by all the participants (subscale categories of FIQ: ability to do various physical activities, ability to work, pain, fatigue, morning stiffness, anxiety and depression) and pretest and posttest bilateral range of motion (ROM) measurements done by a licensed physical therapist assistant.

In addition to the objective assessment using the FIQ and ROM measurements, QOL was also evaluated by collecting qualitative feedback from the participants. The questions on the qualitative feedback form asked the participants to tell us how different components of this exercise program affected their general sense of well-being, pain, stiffness, fatigue, anxiety, ability to do daily activities, self-confidence, aerobic capacity, strength, flexibility, and sleep quality.

Statistical Analysis

Data were analyzed using a one-way ANOVA with repeated measures, multiple comparisons and goodness of fit tests by S-PLUS4 software (MathSoft, Inc., Seattle, WA). The Tukey method was used for multiple comparisons and a one-sample Kolmogorov-Smirnov test of composite normality was performed for the goodness of fit test. The Kruskal-Wallis non-parametric rank sum test for ANOVA was also performed. Statistical significance was set at $p < 0.05$ for all the tests. Descriptive statistics were computed on all the variables in the study.

RESULTS

To be included in the final analysis, the participants were required to be available for all the pretest and the posttest measurements. In addition, a 70% participation rate (14 exercise sessions) was set as the criteria for the participants in the two exercise groups. Twenty-one women met all the completion requirements for the study (retention rate: Total = 69%, C = 67%, G = 100%, H = 40%). There were several reasons given by the women for not completing the study. Busy schedules, family commitments and just being overwhelmed by FM related health problems were the most common reasons given by the four controls that did not complete the post testing and also by five home-based group participants that did not exercise at least fourteen times. One of the home-based participants did not respond to our repeated attempts to contact her. The baseline age (years) means and standard deviations for the participants in the three groups that completed the study are as follows: C = 43.50 ± 11.93 (n = 8), G = 51.78 ± 8.00 (n = 9), H = 56 ± 7.14 (n = 4). The anthropometric data of the research participants is given in Table 2. No injuries resulted from the exercise program during the ten weeks. However, there was one minor flare-up that was reported by the hospital-based subject in the second week of the study.

There were no statistically significant differences between the pretest mean values for the following variables for the three groups: FIQ (P = 0.54), ROM (P = 0.19), TPC (P = 0.06), TPS (P = 0.75). Over the ten-week period, we found significant improvements in the FIQ and the ROM scores of the two exercise groups. However, the TPC and TPS scores did not show any significant improvements (Table 1).

The changes in FIQ scores from pre to post testing were statistically significant (p = 0.0049). The negative values in the FIQ category in Table 1 indicate improvement. The FIQ scores of the hospital based participants and the home based participants changed − 20.84% and − 37.45% respectively. The change in FIQ scores for the control group (−0.18%) was not significant.

For the ROM, the higher posttest scores indicated improvement. The change in ROM mean scores was statistically significant (p = 0.0003). The hospital based participants and the home based participants showed 9.73% and 6.21% improvement in ROM respectively. On the other hand, the control group ROM decreased by − 2.58% during the 10-week period.

The TPC and TPS changes were not statistically significant: TPC (p = 0.8354) and TPS (p = 0.9984). The TPC and TPS scores are presented in Table 1 along with the FIQ and ROM scores for the three groups.

DISCUSSION

The 10-week/20-session Fibromyalgia Exercise Program significantly improved FIQ and ROM of women in two exercise groups compared to the non-exercising control group. However, the TPC and TPS improvements were not statistically significant. In addition to the quantitative data that were collected and analyzed, women in the two exercise groups also provided qualitative feedback. The exercising participants

TABLE 1. Mean scores for the pretest, posttest, change (−), change(−)% mean ± standard deviation for the three groups and the ANOVA p-values for the pre to post changes.

Variables	Groups	Pre	Post	(−) Change	(−) Change % Mean ± SD	(−) P-values
FIQ	Hospital	60.95	48.25	−12.70#	−20.84 ±16.60#	
	Home	50.04	31.30	−18.74#	−37.45 ± 20.09#	0.0049*
	Control	55.99	55.89	−0.10#	−0.18 ± 14.92#	
ROM	Hospital	526.33	577.56	51.22	9.73 ± 4.30	
	Home	551.75	586.00	34.25	6.21 ± 7.32	0.0003*
	Control	575.88	561.00	−14.88	−2.58 ± 4.44	
TPC	Hospital	16.56	16.33	−0.23#	−1.39 ± 13.11#	
	Home	17.50	16.00	−1.50#	−8.57 ± 18.75#	0.8354
	Control	18	17.13	−0.87#	−4.83 ± 11.67#	
TPS	Hospital	42.47	41.50	−0.97#	−2.28 ± 37.33	
	Home	45.88	44.88	−1.00#	−2.18 ± 14.39	0.9984
	Control	47.06	45.81	−1.25#	−2.66 ± 19.81#	

Hospital (n = 9), Home (n = 4), Control (n = 8)
#Negative values show improvement
*indicates p < 0.05

reported self-perceived improvement in general well-being, fatigue, sleep quality, pain, stress, anxiety, self-confidence, strength, aerobic capacity, flexibility, and ability to sit/stand with less pain.

The TPC and TPS results of this study are not consistent with the results of a study done at the Oregon Health Sciences University in Portland, OR (Bennett et al., 1996). Our quantitative analysis combined with the qualitative feedback confirm our theory that the TPC and TPS are effective diagnostic tests but are not very useful for measuring QOL improvements. Since the TPS, and especially the TPC, do not affect patient day-to-day functional ability (and can be very painful tests for the patients), we do not suggest these tests for the purposes of quantifying QOL improvements.

TABLE 2. Anthropometric data of three experimental groups.

	Hospital (G) Weight ± SD	Home (H) Weight ± SD	Control (C) Weight ± SD
Height (inches)	63.88	62.25	64.63
Weight (lbs.) Pre	154.89 ± 40.77	164.75 ± 35.13	146.75 ± 30.18
Weight (lbs.) Post	152.60 ± 38.60	163.92 ± 34.20	145 ± 31.02
BI Fat % Pre	35.00 ± 7.91	40.15 ± 3.78	29.03 ± 11.14
BI Fat % Post	34.23 ± 7.98	39.05 ± 4.28	28.85 ± 11.31
BI Fat (lbs.) Pre	56.50 ± 27.72	67 ± 21.05	45.44 ± 25.65
BI Fat (lbs.) Post	54.89 ± 28.26	64.38 ± 21.59	44.86 ± 25.89

Hospital (n = 9), Home (n = 4), Control (n = 8)

On the other hand, the ROM has a more direct impact on the functional ability. The ROM exercises in this program were designed to effectively stretch and loosen up the tender point locations throughout the body before doing the aerobic and the strengthening exercises. We believe that it is not only the quantity but also the quality of stretching that resulted in minimal post exercise exertion and flare-ups. On several occasions during the course of the study, the participants came to the exercise session in great discomfort, thinking that exercising would be an impossible task that day. But by doing some stretching exercises in a lying down position, they not only got some relief but also renewed their self-confidence. Hence, we conclude that the ROM testing is a good indicator of assessing QOL and the subjective well-being of individuals with FM.

One of the limitations of this study was that there was no random assignment of the subjects to different groups. Furthermore, the group environment and the feedback from the researcher for the hospital-based group may have confounded the claim that the exercises alone produced all the improvements. We believe that for the hospital-based group, having regular interaction and the support of other women with FM for ten weeks was a strong motivator. A non-competitive, supportive group environment setting can be a powerful element in the success of any chronic pain exercise program. The qualitative feedback of the hospital-based group women overwhelmingly supported this conclusion. The constant feedback from the researcher during exercise sessions and, when necessary, minor modifications of the exercises performed clearly contributed to zero percent injury rate and 100% compliance rate for the hospital-based group.

As mentioned earlier, the ten-week period started in October 1999 and concluded in December 1999. The stress associated with the holiday season and the colder weather in December compared to that in October could not be ignored. Because weather changes and stress are known to worsen the FM symptoms, it can be concluded that this exercise program might, in fact, be more effective than the results obtained (Wolfe et al., 1990). Again, the participants reconfirmed this in their qualitative feedback.

The external validity of this research is extremely high. The results can be generalized with confidence to other adult women with FM. Due to the overlapping symptoms of chronic fatigue syndrome (CFS) with FM, there is a possibility that the program may also be beneficial for individuals with CFS (Fulcher & White, 1997; Goldberg, 1989). More research is needed in regard to this question.

The SQ and ICS were used to further understand the impact of FM. All the participants including the controls completed the SQ and ICS. The anxiety, depression, somatization and hostility subscale scores of SQ and the ICS scores for the FM participants were compared with the norms for the normal population (Gandhi, 2000). The women with FM consistently scored higher than their normal counterparts in all these categories. On the other hand for the relaxation, contentment, somatic well-being and friendliness subscales, they consistently scored lower. Every one of the participants in our study had complaints of muscle soreness, stiffness, fatigue and sleep disturbances.

CONCLUSION

The Fibromyalgia Exercise Program described in this article is an effective program in improving QOL of women with FM. It improved QOL of the participants with minimal post-exercise discomfort. The post exercise recovery period would be an important determinant of a long-term adherence to the exercise program. Improved functional ability, general well-being, sleep quality, stress, anxiety, self-confidence, strength, aerobic capacity, flexibility, fatigue and pain were measured with FIQ, ROM and qualitative feedback. Even though the pathophysiology of FM is complex and the clinical research status of FM is in its infancy, our exercise program can be highly effective for improving the QOL. It can also be a useful resource for pain management for women with FM and perhaps for other chronic pain conditions as well.

Implications

This exercise program is a result of years of research and personal experimentation with different types of exercises by the first author. The sequencing of exercises is as important as the percentage of total time spent on different components of the exercise program. The focus needs to be on breathing, relaxation, and stretching exercises and not just the aerobic component. Due to a complex and unique nature of the fibromyalgia syndrome, we strongly suggest that fibromyalgia be addressed as a separate topic for designing exercise programming guidelines. Further research is recommended to explore the benefits of this exercise program as a resource for pain management.

REFERENCES

Abell, N. (1991). The index of clinical stress: A brief measure of subjective stress for practice and research. *Social Work Research and Abstracts, 27*, 12-15.

Bakker, C., Rutten, M., & Santen-Hoeufft, M. (1995). Patient utilities in fibromyalgia and the association with other outcome measures. *Journal of Rheumatology, 22*, 1536-1543.

Bengtsson, A., Backman, E., Lindblom, B., & Skogh, T. (1994). Long term follow-up of fibromyalgia patients: Clinical symptoms, muscular function, laboratory tests–An eight year comparison study. *Journal of Musculoskeletal Pain, 2*, 67-80.

Bennett, R. M. (1994). Exercise and exercise testing in fibromyalgia patients: Lessons learned and suggestions for future studies. *Journal of Musculoskeletal Pain, 2*, 143-152.

Bennett, R. M., Burckhardt, C. S., & Clark, S. R. (1996). Group treatment of fibromyalgia: A six month outpatient program. *Journal of Rheumatology, 23*, 521-528.

Burckhardt, C. S., Clark, S. R. & Bennett, R. M. (1991). The fibromyalgia impact questionnaire: Development and validation. *Journal of Rheumatology, 18*, 728-733.

Burckhardt, C. S., Clark, S. R., & Bennett, R. M. (1993). Fibromyalgia and quality of life: A comparative analysis. *Journal of Rheumatology, 20*, 475-479.

Burckhardt, C. S., Clark, S. R. & Padrick, K. P. (1989). Use of the modified balke treadmill protocol for determining the aerobic capacity of women with fibromyalgia. *Arthritis Care Research, 2*, 165-167.

Burckhardt, C. S., Mannerkorpi, K., Hedenberg, L., & Bjelle, A. (1994). A randomized controlled clinical trial of education and physical training for women with fibromyalgia. *Journal of Rheumatology, 21*, 714-720.

Fulcher, K. Y., & White, P. D. (1997, June). Randomised controlled trial of graded exercise in patients with the chronic fatigue syndrome. *British Medical Journal,* Viridal Duo, http;//www.bmj.com/cgi/content/full/314/7095/1647

Gandhi, N. (2000). Effect of an exercise program on quality of life of women with fibromyalgia. Master's thesis, Washington State University, Pullman.

Goldberg, D. L. (1989). Fibromyalgia and its relation to chronic fatigue syndrome, viral illness and immune abnormalities. *Journal of Rheumatology Supplement, 19,* 91-93.

Henriksson, C. I., Gundmark, A., Benstsson, A., & Ek, A. C. (1992). Living with fibromyalgia. Consequences for everyday life. *Clinical Journal of Pain, 8,* 138-144.

Hiemeyer, K., Lutz, R., & Menninger, H. (1990). Dependence of tender points upon posture–a key to the understanding of fibromyalgia syndrome. *Journal of Manual Medicine, 5,* 169-174.

Kellner, R. (1987). A symptom questionnaire. *Journal of Clinical Psychiatry, 48,* 268-274.

McCain, G. A. (1986). Role of physical fitness training in the fibrositis/fibromyalgia syndrome. *American Journal of Medicine, 81*(3A), 73-77.

McCain, G. A., Bell, D. A., Mai, F. M., & Halliday, P. D. (1988). A controlled study of the effects of a supervised cardiovascular fitness training program on the manifestations of primary fibromyalgia. *Arthritis Rheumatology, 31,* 1135-1141.

Mengshoel, A. M. (1990). Muscle strength and aerobic capacity in primary fibromyalgia. *Clinical and Experimental Rheumatology, 8,* 475-479.

Mengshoel, A. M., Komnaes, H. B., & Forre, O. (1992). The effects of 20 weeks of physical fitness training in female patients with fibromyalgia. *Clinical and Experimental Rheumatology, 10,* 345-349.

Natvig, B., Bruusgaard, D., & Eriksen, W. (1998). Physical leisure activity level and physical fitness among women with fibromyalgia. *Scandanavian Journal of Rheumatology, 27,* 337-341.

Sietsema, K. E., Cooper, D. M., Caro, X., Leibling, R. M., & Louie, S. (1993). Oxygen uptake during exercise in patients with primary fibromyalgia syndrome. *Journal of Rheumatology, 20,* 860-865.

Starlanyl, D., & Copeland, M. E. (1996*). Fibromyalgia and chronic myofascial pain syndrome: A survival manual* (pp. 7-10). Oakland, CA: New Harbinger.

Van Denderen, J. C., Boersma, J. W., Zeinstra, P., Hollander, A. P., & Van Nerbos, B. R. (1992). Physiological effects of exhaustive physical exercise in primary fibromyalgia syndrome (PFS): Is PFS a disorder of neuroendocrine reactivity? *Scandanavian Journal of Rheumatology, 21,* 35-37.

Wolfe, F., Smythe, H. A., & Yunus, M. B. (1990). The American College of Rheumatology 1990 Criteria for the classification of fibromyalgia. *Arthritis Rheumatology, 33*(2),160-172.

Wolfe, R. (1986). The clinical syndrome of fibrositis. *American Journal of Medicine, 81*(3A), 7-13.

Exercise:
Complementary Therapy
for Breast Cancer Rehabilitation

Karen M. Mustian
Jeffrey A. Katula
Diane L. Gill

SUMMARY. Our feminist perspective is one of empowerment for breast cancer survivors, and we believe that physical activity and exercise have the potential to shift the battle away from fear of living to living fully. In light of the psychosocial and cultural factors that influence the interpretation of the breast cancer experience, rehabilitation efforts have shifted from curing the disease to living with the disease, or survival. This shift is reflected in the selection of quality of life as the primary indicant of treatment efficacy. Interpreted from a feminist, empowerment perspective, evidence is presented demonstrating the positive influence of physical activity and exercise on quality of life in breast cancer survivors. We propose that physical activity has the potential to enhance perceptions of capabilities and control, thus empowering the in-

---

Karen M. Mustian, Jeffrey A. Katula, and Diane L. Gill are affiliated with the University of North Carolina at Greensboro.

Address correspondence to: Karen M. Mustian, Department of Exercise and Sport Science, University of North Carolina at Greensboro, P. O. B. 26169, Greensboro, NC 27402-6169 (E-mail: kmmustia@uncg.edu).

[Haworth co-indexing entry note]: "Exercise: Complementary Therapy for Breast Cancer Rehabilitation." Mustian, Karen M., Jeffrey A. Katula, and Diane L. Gill. Co-published simultaneously in *Women & Therapy* (The Haworth Press, Inc.) Vol. 25, No. 2, 2002, pp. 105-118; and: *Exercise and Sport in Feminist Therapy: Constructing Modalities and Assessing Outcomes* (ed: Ruth L. Hall, and Carole A. Oglesby) The Haworth Press, Inc., 2002, pp. 105-118. Single or multiple copies of this article are available for a fee from The Haworth Document Delivery Service [1-800-HAWORTH, 9:00 a.m. - 5:00 p.m. (EST). E-mail address: getinfo@haworthpressinc.com].

105

dividual to create her own reality. We conclude that physical exercise can be a safe and effective complementary and alternative method of therapy for breast cancer survivors. *[Article copies available for a fee from The Haworth Document Delivery Service: 1-800-HAWORTH. E-mail address: <getinfo@haworthpressinc.com> Website: <http://www.HaworthPress.com> © 2002 by The Haworth Press, Inc. All rights reserved.]*

KEYWORDS. Breast cancer, women, exercise, rehabilitation, feminist, alternative treatments

INTRODUCTION

"My wake up call from my healer within came to me through my breasts; I think of it as my 'Amazon awakening.' And so our breasts become a cultural battleground where a war is waged between our fear of living fully and our fear of dying before we've ever lived fully" (Northrup, as cited in Weed, 1996; p. x). Our feminist perspective is one of empowerment for breast cancer survivors, and we believe that physical activity and exercise have the potential to shift the battle away from fear to living fully. When diagnosed with breast cancer, women are faced with a myriad of contemporary and socio-cultural ideologies. Breast cancer survivors are often viewed as victims and subjected to oppressive patriarchal ideologies, including negative stereotypes regarding a lack of femininity and sexuality. These negative stereotypes are grounded in social and cultural interpretations of the side effects resulting from the life saving medical treatments breast cancer survivors currently undergo. Breast cancer survivors routinely lose all or part of their breasts, experience hair loss, weight gain, and early onset menopause. These side effects present psychological, social, and cultural challenges for these women to maintain their feminine and sexual identities. This is particularly true within the Western medical and scientific traditions, which are inherently patriarchal (Keller, 1990). These traditional myopic perspectives of breast cancer stem from an isolated individual focus on disease that fail to consider women's perceptions and the influence of her particular life experience.

It is our position that the phenomenon of breast cancer is significantly influenced by the social and cultural context in which it occurs (Nelson, 1996). As Audre Lorde (1980) eloquently states, "Each woman responds to the crisis that breast cancer brings to her life out of a whole pattern, which is the design of who she is and how her life has been lived. The weave of her everyday existence is the training ground for how she handles crisis" (p. 9). However, Western medical and scientific traditions have predominantly defined the breast cancer experience in terms of the physical body and biomedical outcomes (Friedenreich & Courneya, 1996; Thorne & Murray, 2000). Fortunately, social and cultural interpretations of the breast cancer phenomenon are evolving (Glanz & Lerman, 1992). Most recently, health professionals have embraced a holistic mindset regarding the experience of breast cancer and have adopted biopsychosocial perspectives, as evidenced by the emergence of quality of life as the primary indicant of treatment efficacy. Quality of life can be defined as a multidimensional and complex perceptual concept including many biopsychosocial factors, such as functional ability, psychological functioning, social adjustment, and disease- and treatment-related symptoms (Andersen, Kiecolt-Glaser, & Glaser, 1999). As such, efforts to understand, explain, and treat the phenomenon of breast cancer now incorporate psychological, social, and cultural factors. Consequently, physical activity and exercise have been shown to influence many of these psychosocial factors, which may help move breast cancer rehabilitation from a victim, isolated medical model to a more feminist empowered approach.

In light of this myriad of psychosocial and cultural factors, there is no one stable and absolute reality regarding the breast cancer experience. The individual is an active agent in the construction of her reality, which is created mostly through historical and socio-cultural meanings (Hall, 1996). We base our perspective in social cognitive theory (Bandura, 1986), which posits that humans are active agents in their lives with the power to choose their own behavior and realities. Further, thoughts and actions result from a complex interaction between the individual, environment, and behavior, each of which are reciprocal, fluid, and evolving. Thus, the individual's perception of her constructed reality holds primary importance in determining her quality of life and, therefore, treatment outcome. This is particularly relevant to breast cancer in that individuals may choose to accept dominant patriarchal and socio-culturally constructed stereotypes, involving (non) feminine body-images, sexuality, breast reconstruction, and victimization (e.g., Clark, 1999; Thorne & Murray, 2000) or resist and form positive enabling experiences and environments. It is plausible to suggest that a feminist approach to physical activity may empower survivors with the ability to perceive and create positive, enabling realities.

Research suggests that physical activity and exercise are powerful moderators in the social cognitive model (e.g., Katula, McAuley, Mihalko, & Bane, 1998). For example, it has been demonstrated that even one bout of exercise can enhance women's self-efficacy (i.e., perceptions of their capabilities), the central construct within the social cognitive model (Katula et al., 1998). Furthermore, physical activity and exercise is uniquely situated to positively impact the functional, physical, psychological, and social challenges faced by breast cancer survivors (Courneya & Friedenreich, 1999). Specifically, mastery experiences gained via physical activity and exercise have been shown to positively influence self-perceptions of control and behavior (e.g., McAuley, 1992; Mihalko, McAuley & Bane, 1996). With an increased sense of control, breast cancer survivors may experience an enhanced sense of agency that can empower them to resist dominant patriarchal ideologies and create positive alternative realities as thrivers. Thus, it is important to systematically educate and encourage the increasing number of diverse breast cancer survivors about the benefits of physical activity and exercise in the recovery process.

The American Cancer Society (American Cancer Society, 2000) predicts that approximately 182,800 new cases of breast cancer will be diagnosed during 2001 in the United States, accounting for 30% of all cancer diagnoses in women. Thus, breast cancer is currently the number one diagnosed form of cancer in women. Breast cancer risk increases with age (Kimmick & Muss, 2000), and African American women experience breast cancer less overall than European Americans. However, researchers also report a higher incidence of breast cancer in younger African American women with an age crossover at approximately 50 years. This ultimately results in higher numbers among European Americans (Kerner, Trock, & Mandelblatt, 2000). Additionally, the American Cancer Society (2000) reports that breast cancer rates are lower among Latino and Asian women, with American Indian women experiencing the lowest rate of breast cancer. Furthermore, lesbians may exhibit an increased risk for breast cancer when compared to heterosexual women (Love, 2000).

Moreover, the American Cancer Society (2000) estimates that 41,200 deaths will result from breast cancer and women have a 3% lifetime risk of death from breast cancer. Breast cancer patients of all ages appear to fare similarly well if diagnosis is with localized or regional stages of breast cancer. However, older women are more likely to be diagnosed with metastatic cancer, and possess a higher mortality rate (Kerner, Trock, & Mandelblatt, 2000). Even with the lower incident rates of breast cancer among African American women, their mortality rates are higher than European Americans (Dingnam, 2000; Greenlee, Hill-Harmon, Murrray, & Thun, 2001; Kimmick & Muss, 2000). This constitutes breast cancer as the second largest cause of cancer death among women in the United States (National Cancer Institute, 1998). However, the survival rate of women diagnosed and treated for breast cancer is improving, especially with early detection (Harris, 2000).

Most women diagnosed with breast cancer can expect to live for long periods of time (Rowland & Massie, 2000). The American Cancer Society (2000) reports that the five-year relative survival rate is 96% for women diagnosed with localized breast cancer. The survival rates for women diagnosed with regional and distant metastases are 77% and 21%, respectively, but survival declines after five years (e.g., 10 years, 71%; 15 years, 57%). Improvements in early detection and treatments for breast cancer are responsible for the increased survival rates, and, combined with increased incidence, have resulted in eight million Americans living with a history of cancer (American Cancer Society, 1998). As the number of diverse breast cancer survivors escalates, cancer rehabilitation has become extremely important (Wingo, Tony, & Bolden, 1995) and research focus has shifted from curing the disease to living with the disease and its consequences (Makar, Cumming, Lees, Hundleby, Nabholtz, Kieren, Jenkins, Wentzel, Handman, & Cumming, 1997). Specifically, emphasis has been placed on the quality of life (QOL) concerns of cancer survivors (Bradley & Scharf, 1998; Fawzy, Fawzy, Arndt, & Pasnau, 1995).

It is imperative to understand that unlike treatments for diabetes or heart disease, treatments for cancer are more toxic and intensive (Rowland & Massie, 2000). Breast cancer treatments, such as surgery, chemotherapy, radiotherapy, and pharmaceutical therapy, often result in a host of deleterious side effects that impact several indices of quality of life. Common psychosocial side effects of breast cancer include depression, anxiety, stress, mood disturbances, decreased self-esteem, loss of a sense of control, marital and social withdrawal, poor body image, diminished femininity, self-deprecation, and sexual dysfunction (e.g., Glanz & Lerman, 1992; Penman, Bloom, & Fotopoulos, 1986; Psychological Aspects of Cancer Study Group, 1987; Segar, Katch, Roth, Weinstein, Portner, Glickman, Haslanger, & Wilkins, 1998). Physical and functional side effects of breast cancer include decreased cardiovascular function, diminished strength, decreased pulmonary function, loss of lean body mass, weight change, sleeping difficulty, fatigue, nausea, vomiting, hair loss, osteoporosis, and early onset menopause (e.g., Levine, Raczynski, & Carpenter, 1991; Love, Leventhal, Easterling, & Nerenz, 1989; Segar et al., 1998). Research suggests survivors experience persistent psychosocial distress a year or more after diagnosis (Vinokur, Threatt, Vinokur-Kaplan, & Stariano, 1990). Surprisingly, however, research examining the exact nature of breast cancer quality of life impact is inconsistent (Spencer, Lehman, & Love, 1999).

Some studies have failed to find significant differences between women with and without breast cancer. For example, a recent study compared body esteem in young women with and without breast cancer and found no significant differences (Bello & McIntire, 1995). Indeed, it has even been suggested that breast cancer survival may increase self-esteem and body image (Carpenter, 1997). Furthermore, studies have demonstrated inconsistencies between unidimensional, global, quantitative measures and multidimensional and interpretive process-oriented inquiry concerning breast cancer rehabilitation and quality of life indices, such as self-esteem (e.g., Dibble-Hope, 2000). Although quantitative studies often reveal no differences between breast cancer survivors and asymptomatic counterparts, studies employing qualitative methods indicate significant deleterious effects of breast cancer on quality of life. Thus, the exact nature of breast cancer impact is not well understood and, therefore, traditional rehabilitation methods have not sufficiently addressed the diverse and unique issues faced by breast cancer survivors.

EXERCISE AS COMPLEMENTARY THERAPY

In an effort to mitigate the side effects of cancer and enhance quality of life, many breast cancer patients seek the help of alternative and complementary treatments (VandeCreek, Rogers, & Lester, 1999). Alternative and complementary medical treatment methods have recently become widespread in Western society, which has traditionally embraced only allopathic (Western) medicine (Gevitz, 1996). The National Center for Complementary and Alternative Medicine (NCCAM; Alternative Medicine Report, 1992) classifies complementary and alternative therapies into seven categories: (a) diet and nutrition, (b) mind-body techniques, (c) bioelectromagnetics, (d) traditional and folk remedies, (e) pharmacological and biological treatments, (f) manual healing methods, and (g) herbal medicine. Cassileth and Chapman (1996) report that complementary and alternative methods of treatment (CAM) have received unprecedented use and respectability in recent years. This popularity appears to stem from the demand for a more holistic approach to health care, capable of meeting the complex and dynamic biopsychosocial needs of clients. This seems to be especially true for chronic diseases and diseases involving particularly aggressive treatments, such as cancer. Most patients remain actively engaged in conventional medical therapies while employing the use of CAM of treatment (VandeCreek et al., 1999). Additionally, women from various racial and ethnic groups use CAM of treatment. Lee and colleagues (2000) interviewed Black, Hispanic, Chinese, and White breast cancer survivors and found that half of the women in the study used at least one type of CAM of therapy and one-third used two types of CAM of treatment. Currently, there are a number of CAM of therapy that successfully help individuals cope with breast cancer. These CAM include relaxation training, meditation, social support groups, music therapy, and exercise (e.g., Fawzy et al., 1995).

Physical exercise appears to be particularly suited to address issues faced by breast cancer survivors. More specifically, research suggests that physical activity and exercise reduce a number of negative psychosocial health outcomes, such as depression, anxiety, and stress, and enhance positive outcomes, such as self-esteem, self-efficacy, body image, social physique anxiety, and cognitive function (e.g., Landers & Petruzello, 1994; McAuley, 1994). More importantly, physical activity has been shown to enhance the rehabilitation of individuals with chronic diseases, such as hypertension, cardiovascular disease, diabetes, pulmonary disease, and cancer (e.g., Goldbergh & Elliot, 1994). A plethora of anecdotal reports from clinicians, physical therapists, nurses, and cancer patients themselves exist regarding the benefits of physical activity following cancer diagnosis (e.g., Johnson & Kelly, 1990; Molinaro, Kleinfield, & Lebad, 1986).

With respect to breast cancer survivors, physical activity and exercise has been demonstrated as safe and beneficial during and post allopathic adjuvant therapies (e.g., chemotherapy & radiotherapy). Approximately 26% of the general population use exercise as a CAM of medical treatment (Eisenberg, Kessler, Foster, Norlock, Calkins, & Delbanco, 1993). Relative to breast cancer patients, 76% indicate an interest in exercise as a CAM of treatment, and 38% actually use it. This makes exercise the second most popular complementary and alternative therapy sought and used by breast cancer outpatients (VandeCreek et al., 1999).

A number of studies have demonstrated the effectiveness of various modes of exercise for improving various aspects of quality of life in breast cancer survivors. Several studies have demonstrated that women participating in exercise, such as cycling, walking, and stretching programs (over 2-6 months), while receiving chemotherapy have shown improvements in anxiety, depression, body-image, stress, fatigue, nausea, vomiting, cardiovascular fitness, lean body mass, and weight fluctuation (Dimeo, Stieglitz, Novelli-Fischer, Fetscher, & Keul, 1999; MacVicar & Winningham, 1986; MacVicar, Winningham, & Nickel, 1989; Mock, Burke, Sheehan, Creaton, Winningham, McKenney-Tedder, Schwager, & Lievman, 1994; Winningham, MacVicar, Bondoc, Anderson, & Minton, 1989). Additionally, women have demonstrated improved anxiety, fatigue, physical functioning, and sleeping patterns as a result of participating in walking programs during radiation treatment (Mock, Dow, Meares, Grimm, Dienmann, Haisfield-Wolfe, Quitasol, Mitchell, Chakravarthy, & Gage, 1997). This would suggest that exercise is a safe and potentially invaluable CAM of treatment for breast cancer survivors during traditional adjuvant therapy.

Additionally, women who were post-surgery, chemotherapy, and radiation therapy that participated in a combination of strength training, aquatics, and aerobic exercises (once per week for one month) felt they had gained sufficient physical training, strength, and fighting spirit (Berglund, Bolund, Gustafsson, & Sjoden, 1993). Women participating in Authentic Movement therapy (i.e., dance therapy) who were six months to six years post treatment exhibited improvement in mood (vigor), distress, body image, self-esteem, fatigue, and somatization. They also reported strongly self-perceived improvements in worry, strength, ease, hope, and social support (Dibble-Hope, 2000). Furthermore, studies have demonstrated that women diagnosed within the past year for breast cancer and who exercised generally report better mood (less confusion and more vigor), self-efficacy, self-esteem, and less fatigue than their sedentary cohorts (Baldwin & Courneya, 1997; Carpenter, 1997; Friedenreich & Courneya, 1996; Graydon, Bubela, Irvine, & Vincent, 1995; Pinto & Maruyama, 1999; Young-McCaughan & Sexton, 1991). In fact, as noted previously, Carpenter (1997) suggests that the breast cancer experience may have positive effects on self-esteem and that one of the potential mediators is exercise participation. Thus, exercise participation provides the potential for enhancing psychosocial and physical indices of quality of life empowering breast cancer survivors during and post-treatment.

CONCLUSION

Although we are just beginning to address the quality of life issues faced by breast cancer survivors, physical activity appears to be one form of CAM that may be uniquely suited to address the unique issues faced by survivors. Studies suggest that women diagnosed with breast cancer may exercise safely while under undergoing chemotherapy and radiotherapy. It also appears that exercise is a safe and viable option for these women after high-dose chemotherapy and bone marrow transplants. Furthermore, exercise can be beneficial for many years after diagnosis and throughout the use of pharmaceutical therapy to attenuate the psychosocial and physical sequelae that remain or reoccur for breast cancer survivors. Moreover, physical activity and exercise can be a cost efficient and non-invasive part of breast cancer recovery (Pinto & Maruyama, 1999).

However, most of the women participating in exercise programs following breast cancer diagnosis are self-selected participants (e.g., Baldwin & Courneya, 1997; Carpenter, 1997; Friedenreich & Courneya, 1996; MacVicar et al., 1989; Mock et al., 1994). In other words, they have not been systematically educated and encouraged to participate in physical activity. Indeed, typical post treatment exercise recommendations involve a one-time demonstration of exercises specifically designed to physically rehabilitate damaged muscle tissue, with no attention to quality of life deficits. With the emergence of nationally recognized events involving physical exercise, such as the American Cancer Society's Relay for Life and Reach to Recovery programs, the Susan G. Komen Walk/Runs, and the YMCA Encore programs, the opportunities for women to participate in exercise programs are growing. However, despite documented interest in CAM and exercise, it appears most of these women are still left to seek, discover, and participate in these activities on their own.

Therapists and health professionals may be an important resource about physical activity for breast cancer survivors by providing education and awareness, broader exercise definitions, and follow-up. Therapists can become familiar with nationally recognized physical activity programs that are offered specifically for breast cancer survivors, such as the aforementioned American Cancer Society's Reach to Recovery program and Relay for Life events, the Susan G. Komen walk/run, and the YMCA's Encore program. Additionally, many local hospitals and cancer centers are beginning to offer physical exercise programs for breast cancer survivors. Furthermore, it is imperative that therapists and social workers familiarize themselves with the safety guidelines for participation in physical activity developed by the American College of Sports Medicine and the Physical Therapy Association. With this information, therapists can empower clients and help to raise awareness concerning the benefits of exercise for breast cancer survivors. Therapists can also assist clients in creating a broad definition of exercise that incorporates many forms of physical activity. Most importantly, therapists can encourage breast cancer survivors to define physical activity and exercise in a manner that is consistent with their individual social and cultural identity. For some women, this might involve participating in traditional forms of exercise, such as walking, jogging, swimming, and weight training. Other breast cancer survivors may find it more appealing to participate in alternative forms of physical activity, such as yoga, tai chi, chi kung, or dance therapy. Furthermore, breast cancer survivors may realize the value of adopting a physically active lifestyle, which may include activities such as walking the dog, gardening, and moderate to vigorous household activities. Lastly, therapists can provide a systematic follow-up for breast cancer survivors regarding physical activity and exercise participation. This could be done in several ways, such as individual appointment sessions, support group meetings, journaling or telephone/electronic contact.

It should be noted that therapists must be acutely aware of the potential dangers and limitations inherent in prescribing physical activity and exercise for breast cancer survivors. For example, although evidence is scarce, it has been suggested that physical exercise can increase one's risk for lymphadema, a pooling of lymphatic fluids in the arm that can be quite harmful (Pinto & Maruyama, 1999). Additionally, the optimal mode, frequency, intensity, and duration of exercise required to maximize quality of life benefits in breast cancer survivors is not known. Finally, breast cancer survivors feeling disconnected from their bodies may be reluctant if not averse to performing physical activity in the face of the social evaluation inherent in contemporary and traditional exercise settings. Therefore, motivation and exercise adherence will most likely be a barrier. However, these barriers can be overcome within a feminist empowerment approach to exercise and breast cancer recovery.

In summary, physical activity and exercise can be a safe complementary therapy for breast cancer survivors during and post adjuvant therapy. Moreover, a lifestyle approach to exercise participation with consideration of each woman's unique cultural and social situation can facilitate a sense of agency in women diagnosed with breast cancer. Active women gain competence and control, and become confident and empowered to move beyond oppressive, patriarchal ideologies regarding the breast cancer experience. This empowerment allows them to create alternative realities that enable them to thrive throughout the duration of their illness and recovery resulting in a full, active life. In closing, "Breast cancer is a dance of initiation, for no woman who dances with cancer is ever the same. She has visited the source and tasted the waters of life and death, savored the sweetness and the sharpness of her own mortality, and tasted her desire to survive" (Weed, 1996; p. xiii).

REFERENCES

Alternative Medicine: Expanding Medical Horizons. (1992). *A Report to the National Institutes of Health on Alternative Medical Systems and Practices in the United States*. Washington, DC: US Government Printing Office.

American Cancer Society. (1998). *Cancer facts and figures*. Atlanta, GA: American Cancer Society.

American Cancer Society. (2000). *Cancer facts and figures: Breast cancer*. [On-line]. Available: http://www3.cancer.org/cancerinfo/sitecenter.asp?ct=1&ctid=8&scp=8.3.2.40030&scs=4&scss=1&scdoc=42000&pnt=2&language=english.

Andersen, B. L., Kiecolt-Glaser, J. K., & Glaser, R. (1999). A biobehavioral model of cancer stress and disease course. In R. M. Suinn & G. R. Vandenbos (Eds.), *Cancer Patients and Their Families* (pp. 3-32). Washington, DC: American Psychological Association.

Baldwin, M. K., & Courneya, K. S. (1997). Exercise and self-esteem in breast cancer survivors: An application of the exercise and self-esteem model. *Journal of Sport & Exercise Psychology, 19*, 347-358.

Bandura, A. (1997). *Self-efficacy: The exercise of control*. New York, NY: W. H. Freeman Company.

Bello, L. K. & McIntire, S. N. (1995). Body image disturbances in young adults with cancer. *Cancer Nursing, 18*(2), 138-143.

Berglund, G., Bolund, C., Gustafsson, U., & Sjoden, P. (1993). Starting Again–A comparison study of a group rehabilitation program for cancer patients. *Acta Oncology, 32*, 15-21.

Bradley, P. & Scharf, M. (1998). Getting connected: African-Americans living beyond breast cancer. Ardmore, PA: Living Beyond Breast Cancer.

Carpenter, J. S. (1997). Self-esteem and well being among women with breast cancer and women in an age-matched comparison group. *Journal of Psychosocial Oncology, 15*(3/4), 59-81.

Cassileth, B. & Chapman, C. (1996). Alternative cancer medicine: A ten-year update. *Cancer Invest. 14*(4), 396-404.

Clark, J. N. (1999). Breast cancer in mass circulating magazines in the U.S.A. and Canada, 1974-1995. *Women & Health, 28*(4), 113-130.

Courneya, K. S. & Friedenreich, C. M. (1999). Physical exercise and quality of life following cancer diagnosis: A literature review. *Annals of Behavioral Medicine, 21*(2), 171-179.

Dibble-Hope, S. (2000). The use of dance/movement therapy in psychological adaptation to breast cancer. *The Arts in Psychotherapy, 27*(1), 51-68.

Dimeo, F. C., Stieglitz, R. D., Novelli-Fischer, U., Fetscher, S., & Keul, J. (1999). Effects of physical activity on the fatigue and psychologic status of cancer patients during chemotherapy. *Cancer, 85*(10), 2273-2277.

Dingnam, J. J. (2000). Differences in breast cancer prognosis among African American and Caucasian women. *CA: A Cancer Journal for Clinicians, 50*, 50-64.

Eisenberg, D., Kessler, R., Foster, C., Norlock, F., Calkins, D., & Delbanco, T. (1993). Unconventional medicine in the United States: Prevalence, costs, and patterns of use. *New England Journal of Medicine, 328*, 246–252.

Fawzy, F. I., Fawzy, N. W., Arndt, L. A., & Pasnau, R. O. (1995). Critical review of psychosocial interventions in cancer care. *Archives of General Psychiatry, 52*, 100-113.

Friedenreich, C. M. & Courneya, K. S. (1996). Exercise as rehabilitation for cancer patients. *Clinical Journal of Sport Medicine, 6*, 237-244.

Glanz, K. & Lerman, C. (1992). Psychosocial impact of breast cancer: A critical review. *Annals of Behavioral Medicine, 14*, 204-210.

Gevitz, N. (1996). The scope and challenge of unconventional medicine. *Advances, 9*(3), 4-11.

Goldbergh, L. & Elliot, D. L. (1994). *Exercise for prevention and treatment of illness.* Philadelphia, PA: F. A. Davis Company.

Graydon, J. E., Bubela, N., Irvine, D., & Vincent, L. (1995). Fatigue-reducing strategies used by patients receiving treatment for cancer. *Cancer Nursing, 18*, 23-28.

Greenlee, Hill-Harmon, Murray, & Thun. (2001). *CA: A Cancer Journal for Clinicians, 51*, 15-36.

Hall, M. A. (1996). *Feminism and sporting bodies.* Champaign, IL: Human Kinetics.

Harris, J. R. (2000). Staging of breast carcinoma. In J. R. Harris, M. E. Lippman, M. Morrow, & S. Hellman (Eds.), *Diseases of the breast* (pp. 457-459). Philadelphia: Lippincott-Raven.

Johnson, J. B. & Kelly, A. W. (1990). A multifaceted rehabilitation program for women with cancer. *Oncology Nursing Forum, 17*, 691-695.

Katula, J., McAuley, E., Mihalko, S., & Bane, S. (1998). Mirror, mirror on the wall . . . exercise environment influences on self-efficacy. *Journal of Social Behavior & Personality, 13*(2), 319-332.

Keller, E. F. (1990). Gender and Science. In J. Nielsen (Ed.), *Feminist research methods* (pp. 41-57). Boulder, CO: Westview Press.

Kerner, J. F., Trock, B. J., & Mandelblatt, J. S. (2000). Breast cancer in minority women. In J. R. Harris, M. E. Lippman, M. Morrow, & S. Hellman (Eds.), *Diseases of the breast* (pp. 955-966). Philadelphia: Lippincott-Raven.

Kimmick, G. G., & Muss, H. B. (2000). Breast cancer in minority women. In J. R. Harris, M. E. Lippman, M. Morrow, & S. Hellman (Eds.), *Diseases of the breast* (pp. 945-954). Philadelphia: Lippincott-Raven.

Landers, D. M. & Petruzzello, S. J. (1994). Physical activity, fitness, and anxiety. In C. Bouchard, R. J. Shepard, & T. Stephens (Eds.), *Physical Activity, Fitness, and Health–International Proceedings and Consensus Statement* (pp. 868-882). Champaign, IL: Human Kinetics.

Lee, M. M., Lin, S. S., Wrensch, M. R., Adler, S. R., & Eisenberg. (2000). Alternative therapies used by women with breast cancer in four ethnic populations. *Journal of the National Cancer Institute, 92*(1), 42-47.

Levine, E. G., Raczynski, J. M., & Carpenter, J. T. (1991). Weight gain with breast cancer adjuvant treatment. *Cancer, 67*, 1954-1959.

Lorde, A. (1980). *The cancer journals*. San Francisco, CA: Aunt Lute Books.

Love, S. M. (2000). *Dr. Susan Love's Breast Book*. New York, NY: Pereus Publishing.

Love, R. R., Leventhal, H., Easterling, D. V., & Nerenz, D. R. (1989). Side effects and emotional distress during cancer chemotherapy. *Cancer, 63*, 604-612.

MacVicar, M. G. & Winningham, M. L. (1986). Promoting the functional capacity of cancer patients. *Cancer Bulletin, 38*, 235-239.

MacVicar, M. G., Winningham, M. L., & Nickel, J. L. (1989). Effects of aerobic interval training on cancer patients' functional capacity. *Nursing Research, 38*, 348-351.

Makar, K., Cumming, C. E., Lees, A. W., Hundleby, M., Nabholtz, J. M., Kieren, D. K., Jenkins, H., Wentzel, C., Handman, M., & Cumming, D. C. (1997). Sexuality, body image and quality of life after high dose or conventional chemotherapy for metastatic breast cancer. *Canadian Journal of Human Sexuality, 6*, 1-8.

McAuley, E. (1992). Understanding exercise behavior: A self-efficacy perspective. In G. C. Roberts (Ed.) *Motivation in Sport and Exercise* (pp. 107-127). Champaign, IL: Human Kinetics.

McAuley, E. (1994). Self-efficacy and intrinsic motivation in exercising middle-aged adults. *Journal of Applied Gerontology, 13*(4), 355-376.

Meyer, T. J., & Mark, M. M. (1995). Effects of psychosocial interventions with adult cancer patients: A meta-analysis of randomized experiments. *Health Psychology, 14*, 101-108.

Milhalko, S. L., McAuley, E., & Bane, S. M. (1996). Self-Efficacy and affective responses to acute exercise in middle-aged adults. *Journal of Social Behavior and Personality, 11*(2), 375-385.

Mock, V., Burke, M. B., Sheehan, P., Creaton, E. M., Winningham, M. L., McKenney-Tedder, S., Schwager, L. P., & Liebman, M. (1994). A nursing program for women with breast cancer receiving adjuvant chemotherapy. *Oncology Nursing Forum, 21*(5), 899-907.

Mock, V., Dow, K. H., Meares, C. J., Grimm, P. M., Dienmann, J. A., Haisfield-Wolfe, M. E., Quitasol, W., Mitchell, S., Chakravarthy, A., & Gage, I. (1997). Effects of exercise on fatigue, physical functioning, and emotional distress during radiation therapy for breast cancer. *Oncology Nursing Forum, 24*(6), 991-1000.

Molinaro, J., Kleinfeld, M., & Lebed, S. (1986). Management of breast cancer: A clinical report. *Physical Therapy, 66*, 967-969.

National Cancer Institute. (1998). *SEER cancer statistics review, 1973-1995*. Bethesda, MD: National Center for Health Statistics.

Nelson, J. P. (1996). Struggling to gain meaning: Living with the uncertainty of breast cancer. *Advances in Nursing Science, 18*(3), 59-76.

Penman, D. T., Bloom, J. R., & Fotopoulos, S. (1986). The impact of mastectomy on self-concept and social function: A combined cross-sectional and longitudinal study with comparison groups. *Women & Health, 11*(3-4), 101-130.

Pinto, B. M. & Maruyama, N. C. (1999). Exercise in the rehabilitation of breast cancer survivors. *Psycho-oncology, 8*, 191-206.

Psychological Aspects of Breast Cancer Study Group. (1987). Psychological response to mastectomy: A prospective comparison study. *Cancer, 59*, 189-196.

Rowland, J. H. & Massie, M. J. (2000). Breast cancer in minority women. In J. R. Harris, M. E. Lippman, M. Morrow, & S. Hellman (Eds.), *Diseases of the breast* (pp. 1009-1031). Philadelphia, PA: Lippincott-Raven.

Segar, M. L., Katch, V. L., Roth, R. S., Weinstein, A. G., Portner, T. I., Glickman, S. G., Haslanger, S., & Wilkins, E. G. (1998). The effect of aerobic exercise on self-esteem and depressive and anxiety symptoms among breast cancer survivors. *Oncology Nursing Forum, 25*(1), 107-113.

Spencer, S. M., Lehman, J. M., & Love, N. (1999). Concerns about breast cancer and relations to psychosocial well being in a multiethnic sample of early-stage patients. *Health Psychology, 18*, 159-168.

Thorne, S. E. & Murray, C. (2000). Social constructions of breast cancer. *Health Care for Women International, 11*, 141-159.

VandeCreek, L., Rogers, E., & Lester, J. (1999). Use of alternative therapies among breast cancer outpatients compared with the general population. *Alternative Therapies, 5*(1), 71-76.

Vinokur, A. D., Threatt, B. A., Vinokur-Kaplan, D., & Stariano, W. A. (1990). The process of recovery from breast cancer for younger and older patients: Changes during the first year. *Cancer, 65*, 1242-1254.

Weed, S. S. (1996). *Breast cancer? Breast health! The wise woman way.* Woodstock, NY: Ash Tree Publishing.

Wingo, P. A., Tony, T., & Bolden, S. (1995). Cancer statistics, 1995. *A Cancer Journal for Clinicians, 45*(1), 8-30.

Winningham, M. L., MacVicar, M. G., Bondoc, M., Anderson, J. I., & Minton, J. P. (1989). Effect of aerobic exercise on body weight and composition in patients with breast cancer on adjuvant chemotherapy. *Oncology Nursing Forum, 16*, 683-689.

Young-McCaughan, S., & Sexton, D. L. (1991). A retrospective investigation of the relationship between aerobic exercise and quality of life in women with breast cancer. *Oncology Nursing Forum, 18*, 751-757.

Jewish Women in Therapy: Seen But Not Heard, edited by Rachel Josefowitz Siegel, MSW, and Ellen Cole, PhD (Vol. 10, No. 4, 1991). *"A varied collection of prose and poetry, first-person stories, and accessible theoretical pieces that can help Jews and non-Jews, women and men, therapists and patients, and general readers to grapple with questions of Jewish women's identities and diversity." (Canadian Psychology)*

Women's Mental Health in Africa, edited by Esther D. Rothblum, PhD, and Ellen Cole, PhD (Vol. 10, No. 3, 1990). *"A valuable contribution and will be of particular interest to scholars in women's studies, mental health, and cross-cultural psychology." (Contemporary Psychology)*

Motherhood: A Feminist Perspective, edited by Jane Price Knowles, MD, and Ellen Cole, PhD (Vol. 10, No. 1/2, 1990). *"Provides some enlightening perspectives. . . . It is worth the time of both male and female readers." (Contemporary Psychology)*

Diversity and Complexity in Feminist Therapy, edited by Laura Brown, PhD, ABPP, and Maria P. P. Root, PhD (Vol. 9, No. 1/2, 1990). *"A most convincing discussion and illustration of the importance of adopting a multicultural perspective for theory building in feminist therapy. . . . This book is a must for therapists and should be included on psychology of women syllabi." (Association for Women in Psychology Newsletter)*

Fat Oppression and Psychotherapy, edited by Laura S. Brown, PhD, and Esther D. Rothblum, PhD (Vol. 8, No. 3, 1990). *"Challenges many traditional beliefs about being fat . . . A refreshing new perspective for approaching and thinking about issues related to weight." (Association for Women in Psychology Newsletter)*

Lesbianism: Affirming Nontraditional Roles, edited by Esther D. Rothblum, PhD, and Ellen Cole, PhD (Vol. 8, No. 1/2, 1989). *"Touches on many of the most significant issues brought before therapists today." (Newsletter of the Association of Gay & Lesbian Psychiatrists)*

Women and Sex Therapy: Closing the Circle of Sexual Knowledge, edited by Ellen Cole, PhD, and Esther D. Rothblum, PhD (Vol. 7, No. 2/3, 1989). *"Adds immeasureably to the feminist therapy literature that dispels male paradigms of pathology with regard to women." (Journal of Sex Education & Therapy)*

The Politics of Race and Gender in Therapy, edited by Lenora Fulani, PhD (Vol. 6, No. 4, 1988). *Women of color examine newer therapies that encourage them to develop their historical identity.*

Treating Women's Fear of Failure, edited by Esther D. Rothblum, PhD, and Ellen Cole, PhD (Vol. 6, No. 3, 1988). *"Should be recommended reading for all mental health professionals, social workers, educators, and vocational counselors who work with women." (The Journal of Clinical Psychiatry)*

Women, Power, and Therapy: Issues for Women, edited by Marjorie Braude, MD (Vol. 6, No. 1/2, 1987). *"Raise[s] therapists' consciousness about the importance of considering gender-based power in therapy . . . welcome contribution." (Australian Journal of Psychology)*

Dynamics of Feminist Therapy, edited by Doris Howard (Vol. 5, No. 2/3, 1987). *"A comprehensive treatment of an important and vexing subject." (Australian Journal of Sex, Marriage and Family)*

A Woman's Recovery from the Trauma of War: Twelve Responses from Feminist Therapists and Activists, edited by Esther D. Rothblum, PhD, and Ellen Cole, PhD (Vol. 5, No. 1, 1986). *"A milestone. In it, twelve women pay very close attention to a woman who has been deeply wounded by war." (The World)*

Women and Mental Health: New Directions for Change, edited by Carol T. Mowbray, PhD, Susan Lanir, MA, and Marilyn Hulce, MSW, ACSW (Vol. 3, No. 3/4, 1985). *"The overview of sex differences in disorders is clear and sensitive, as is the review of sexual exploitation of clients by therapists. . . . Mandatory reading for all therapists who work with women." (British Journal of Medical Psychology and The British Psychological Society)*

Women Changing Therapy: New Assessments, Values, and Strategies in Feminist Therapy, edited by Joan Hamerman Robbins and Rachel Josefowitz Siegel, MSW (Vol. 2, No. 2/3, 1983). *"An excellent collection to use in teaching therapists that reflection and resolution in treatment do not simply lead to adaptation, but to an active inner process of judging." (News for Women in Psychiatry)*

Current Feminist Issues in Psychotherapy, edited by The New England Association for Women in Psychology (Vol. 1, No. 3, 1983). *Addresses depression, displaced homemakers, sibling incest, and body image from a feminist perspective.*

Index

Feeling Good exercises, 34
Feminist therapy
    consciousness raising in, 11
    defined, 10
    defining principles of, 11
    described, 10-11
    empowerment in, 11,14
    goals of, exercise as contribution
        to, 9-22. *See also* Exercise,
        and feminist therapy
    personal is political in, 14
Fibromyalgia
    characteristics of, 92-93
    defined, 92
    exercise program effects on
        quality of life of women
        with, 91-103
    study of
        design of, 94-95
        discussion of, 98-101
        implications of, 102
        index of clinical stress in, 96
        introduction to, 92-93
        Kolmogorov-Smirnov test
            in, 97
        Kruskal-Wallis non-
            parametric rank
            sum test of
            ANOVA in, 97
        materials/assessment
            instruments in,
            95-97
        method of, 93-97
        participants in, 93-94
        procedure/exercise
            program, 94-95
        quality-of-life assessment
            in, 97
        range of motion
            measurement in, 96
        results of, 97-98,99t
        statistical analysis in, 97
        symptom questionnaire in, 96
        tender point count
            assessment in, 96

    tender point severity in, 96
    inactivity due to, deconditioning
        resulting from, 93
    musculoskeletal pain due to, 92
    prevalence of, 92
Fibromyalgia Impact Questionnaire
    (FIQ), 93-94,95-96,97
FIG. *See* Fibromyalgia Impact
    Questionnaire (FIQ)
Fight-or-flight pattern, organizing
    women's physical activity to
    accommodate, 87-89
Fight-or-flight stress response model, 78
FIQ. *See* Fibromyalgia Impact
    Questionnaire (FIQ)
First Tee, 85
Freedman, J., 68
Freson, T., 91

Gaertner, S.L.
Game(s), and movement, 49-51
Gandhi, N., 91
Gender, as factor in women's mental
    health challenges, 1
Genogram(s), Sport/Exercise/Movement
    in assessment of familial influence,
    47-48
    discussion of, 48-49
Gill, D.L., 105
Griest, J.H., 44
Gritman Medical Center, 94-95
Group therapy, for women with chronic
    mental illness, exercise and
    movement as adjunct to, 39-55.
    See also Exercise, and
    movement, as adjunct to group
    therapy for women with
    chronic mental illness
Grove City v. Bell Supreme Court
    decision, 12-13
Gruenewald, T., 76
Gullo, K., 29
Gurung, R., 76

For Product Safety Concerns and Information please contact our
EU representative GPSR@taylorandfrancis.com Taylor & Francis
Verlag GmbH, Kaufingerstraße 24, 80331 München, Germany